Be You

Advanced Kundalini Yoga Kriyas from the late '90s

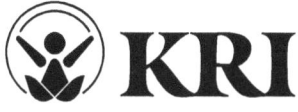

A KUNDALINI RESEARCH INSTITUTE PUBLICATION

Kundalini Yoga as taught by Yogi Bhajan

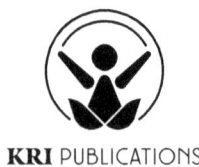

KRI PUBLICATIONS

© 2025 KUNDALINI RESEARCH INSTITUTE
PUBLISHED BY THE KUNDALINI RESEARCH INSTITUTE
TRAINING • PUBLISHING • RESEARCH • RESOURCES
PO BOX 1819
SANTA CRUZ, NM 87532
WWW.KUNDALINIRESEARCHINSTITUTE.ORG
ISBN: ISBN 979-8-9886160-5-4

MANAGING EDITOR: MARIANA LAGE (HARISHABAD KAUR)
CONSULTING EDITOR: AMRIT SINGH KHALSA, PHD
COVER, CREATIVE CONCEPT AND LAYOUT: FERNANDA MONTE-MOR
ILLUSTRATOR: JANIS SOUZA
REVIEWER: SIRI NEEL KAUR KHALSA, DIANA NANU AND LIV DHYAN KAUR
PROOFREADING: CARLOS ANDREI SIQUARA
EDITORIAL ASSISTANT: ANTONIO LARA SILVA

© **Kundalini Research Institute.** All teachings, yoga sets, techniques, kriyas and meditations courtesy of The Teachings of Yogi Bhajan. Reprinted with permission. Unauthorized duplication is a violation of applicable laws. ALL RIGHTS RESERVED. No part of these Teachings may be reproduced or transmitted in any form by any means, electronic or mechanical, including photocopying and recording, or by any information storage and retrieval system, except as may be expressly permitted in writing by The Teachings of Yogi Bhajan. To request permission, please write to KRI at PO Box 1819, Santa Cruz, NM 87567 or see www.kundaliniresearchinstitute.org.

The diet, exercise and lifestyle suggestions in this book come from ancient yogic traditions. Nothing in this book should be construed as medical advice. Neither the author nor the publisher shall be liable or responsible for any loss, injury, damage, allegedly arising from any information or suggestion in this book. The benefits attributed to the practice of Kundalini Yoga and meditation stem from centuries-old yogic tradition. Results will vary with individuals. Always check with your personal physician or licensed care practitioner before making any significant modification in your diet or lifestyle to ensure that the routine changes are appropriate for your personal health condition and consistent with any medication you may be taking.

This publication has received the KRI Seal of Approval. This Seal is given only to products that have been reviewed for accuracy and integrity of the sections containing the 3HO lifestyle and Kundalini Yoga as taught by Yogi Bhajan®. For more information about Kundalini Yoga as taught by Yogi Bhajan® please see **www.kundaliniresearchinstitute.org.**

TABLE OF CONTENTS
—

INTRODUCTION 7
    Before You Begin 10

ADVANCED KUNDALINI YOGA KRIYAS
FROM THE LATE '90S 13

1 / Free Earthly Attachment and Give God a Chance 14
2 / Tuning Up the Frontal Lobe 16
3 / Meditation for Applied Consciousness 18
4 / Meditation for Inner Strength and Balance 20
5 / Expand to Create Momentum 22
6 / Meditation in Action 28
7 / Shine Your Ligh 30
8 / Meditation to Become Divine 32
9 / Raise Your Vibration to Heal Others 34
10 / See With An Infinite Perspective 36
11 / Become Sensitive and Alert 38
12 / Make Progress in Life 42
13 / Creative Thought and Action for Success 44
14 / Access Reserve Strength to Confront Reality 46
15 / Kriya to Recognize the God Within 52
16 / Create a Beam for Opportunity 58
17 / Come Into Oneness 64

18 /	Reserve Energy to Build Stature	68
19 /	Experience God Within and Find Contentment	70
20 /	Open the Heart to Experience Yourself	74
21 /	Open the Heart Center and See Life as a Gift	77
22 /	For Clarity of Mind	80
23 /	Meditation for Subtlety and Intuition	84
24 /	Control Your Thoughts	86
25 /	Energize the Brain	88
26 /	Change Your Electromagnetic Field	90
27 /	Resolve Inner Anger To Be Happy	92
28 /	Flow of Prosperityt	94
29 /	Bless All Beingst	96
30 /	Forgive to Be Authentic and Honest	98
31 /	Meditation for Manifestation	100
32 /	Be Your True Self	102
33 /	Resolve Anger for Inner Balance	104
34 /	Let Go of Self-Judgment	106
35 /	Use Shabad to Know Your Impact	108
36 /	Conquer Inner Anger and Burn it Out	111
37 /	Releasing Childhood Anger	113
38 /	Trust God To Pave The Way	114
39 /	Experience Interconnectedness	118
40 /	Use Your Energy to Live Your Own Truth	123
41 /	Become Vast and Open to Everything	124
42 /	Kriya To Reveal the Core Reality of You	126

43 /	Expand Into Your Excellence	130
44 /	Naad Sutra Kriya	136
45 /	To Act From the Vastness of Your Heart	138
46 /	Kriya to Awaken Intuition	140
47 /	Kriya To Increase Circulation and Energize The Brain	144
48 /	Kriya to Develop Grit and Grace	146
49 /	Be Yourself Meditation	150
50 /	Kriya To Trust Yourself	152
51 /	Know Yourself to Become a Leader	154
52 /	Meditation to See All Life as a Blessing	156
53 /	For a Golden Aura	158
54 /	Face Yourself and Relax	160
55 /	Know Yourself and Conduct Yourself	164

INTRODUCTION
—

It is with immense joy and gratitude that we present *Be You: Advanced Kundalini Yoga Kriyas from the late '90s*, a collection of powerful, unpublished kriyas that guide you to embrace authenticity, self-awareness, and inner peace through recognizing the divine within.

This manual is a testament to the enduring wisdom and transformative potential of Kundalini Yoga. It is designed for dedicated practitioners, yoga teachers, and teacher trainers who are committed to deepening their practice and expanding their consciousness. Within these pages, you will find 55 advanced, multi-exercise meditation kriyas, deeply engaging through intense breathing, arm postures, navel work, and a lot of mantra chanting. These practices are intended to empower you, build confidence, and fortify your self-power.

The journey of this publication begins with a student's request to make a short selection of Yogi Bhajan's lectures publicly accessible through the Library of Teachings. Amrit Singh and Nirvair Singh took on the task of reviewing these lectures and practicing from them. Inspired by their experiences, Amrit proposed integrating these initial 20 practices into a new book. This initiative evolved through meticulous selection and practice, focusing on lectures and classes from July 1998 to June 1999. We went through the classes from this twelve-month period and decided to include all meditations, excluding Master's Touch classes, Khalsa Women's Training Camp classes (KWTC), and Healers Course classes. In this process, we carefully curated 55 practices, with only five being previously published in a KRI book. Finally, we have this final selection of wonderful and powerful practices that touch on the theme of being yourself and nurturing your higher Self.

As we worked on the write-ups and the accuracy process, we continually remembered Yogi Bhajan's teachings on patience, dwelling in God, and the importance of being true to oneself. In a world where we often find ourselves caught in an unconscious web of comparison and competition, these meditation kriyas serve as a vital reminder to stay connected to our inner selves and trust that the Universe will provide for us as long as we are our own singular selves.

But to be our true selves, we need to know ourselves. The practices encourage us to cultivate a daily spiritual practice, grounding us in the present moment and fostering a deep awareness of our body, mind, and spirit. In this process, it's of high importance to recognize our mental patterns, get rid of fears and doubts, and dissolve inner anger. As Yogi Bhajan taught us in that famous saying about how patience pays: "You need a million things. Millions of things will reach you if you are stable, established, firm, patient."

We can go for different spiritual traditions, and most of them, if not all, will teach us that the basic daily spiritual practice is to stay present in the here and now, awake and aware. This basic practice, although simple, holds the key to knowing ourselves. Thus, practicing mindfulness, or, in other words, applying our meditative mind to our daily lives, leads us to self-awareness and our own authenticity, which brings abundance, health, and wellbeing. By nurturing our higher selves and embodying our true nature, we can positively impact and help others, extending the light of our practice into the world.

You'll notice that one of the recurring concepts in these meditations is the pivotal role of the mind. For instance, "Tuning Up the Frontal Lobe" and "Meditation for Applied Consciousness" both emphasize the need to transcend duality and karma by acting from a meditative mind. This dharmic living—rooted in a unified, meditative state—fosters actions that align with our true selves, devoid of the consequences that arise from duality.

Additionally, "Meditation for Inner Strength and Balance" and "Raise Your Vibration to Heal Others" illustrate how breathwork and meditation can cultivate mental steadiness and a balanced psyche. These, as well as other practices, help us respond to life's challenges from a place of inner strength rather than reactivity. As a steady mind is important, so is an open heart to holding self-awareness in daily life. When we operate from our liberated heart centers, we naturally exhibit compassion, calmness, kindness, and authenticity in our interactions.

Self-discipline is another key aspect highlighted in practices such as "Expand Into Your Excellence" and "Kriya to Develop Grit and Grace." These meditations underscore the importance of consistent discipline in living authentically.

Self-discipline not only enhances our personal growth but also empowers us to communicate and act from a place of integrity and grace.

Other practices throughout the book remind us to meditate on Infinity and view life through our subtle awareness so that we can transcend our limited perspectives and recognize our intrinsic value and light. This broader awareness helps us understand that all experiences are part of a divine play, fostering a sense of peace and acceptance. In other words, by dwelling in God and befriending our souls, we align with our true selves and embrace the fullness of our being.

In a nutshell, the essence of these kriyas is to help you tap into your creative consciousness and develop a character that reflects your true self. By engaging your neutral, intuitive, and meditative mind and by opening your heart center, you can dissolve inner anger, access your reserve energy, and know your inner strength. This, in turn, enables you to recognize and feel the divine within, enhancing your self-worth and self-trust.

We hope that *Be You: Advanced Kundalini Yoga Kriyas from the late '90s* will be a valuable resource on your journey towards self-discovery and spiritual growth. May these teachings inspire you to live authentically and fully, recognizing your light within yourself and in all those around you.

**Mariana Lage
(HariShabad Kaur Khalsa)**
KRI Publishing Manager

Before You Begin

If you're new to Kundalini Yoga, note that it's always a good practice to tune in before you begin your yoga each day. Here, we share key points to be aware of when doing the practices below.

TUNING IN

Every Kundalini Yoga session begins with chanting the Adi Mantra[1], "Ong Namo Guru Dev Namo." By chanting it with the right pronunciation and projection, the student becomes open to their higher self, the source of all guidance, and accesses the protective link between himself or herself and the consciousness of the divine teacher.

Sit in a comfortable cross-legged position with the spine straight. Place the palms of the hands together as if in prayer, with the fingers pointing straight up, and then press the joints of the thumbs into the center of the chest at the sternum. Inhale deeply. Focus your concentration on the Third Eye Point. As you exhale, chant the entire mantra in one breath. If you can't chant on a single breath, then take a quick sip of air through the mouth after "Ong Namo" and then chant the rest of the mantra, extending the sound as long as possible. As you chant "Ong," let the sound vibrate the inner chambers of the sinuses and the upper palate to create a mild pressure at the Third Eye Point. The mouth is slightly open, and the lips held firm, increasing the resonance while the sound comes out through the nose. The sound "Dev" is chanted a minor third higher than the other sounds of the mantra. Chant this mantra at least three times before beginning your Kundalini Yoga practice.

The "O" sound in Ong is long, as in "go," and of short duration. The "ng" sound is long and produces a definite vibration on the roof of the mouth and the cranium. The "O," as in "go," is held longer. The first syllable of Guru is pronounced as in the word "good." The second syllable rhymes with "true." The first syllable is short, and the second one is long. The word Dev rhymes with "gave."

"Ong" is the infinite creative energy experienced in manifestation and activity. It is a variant of the cosmic syllable "Om," which refers to God in its absolute or

---

1 "Adi" means primal or first. Thus, Adi Mantra is the first, or primal, mantra.

unmanifest state. "Namo" has the same root as the Sanskrit word "Namaste," which means reverent greetings. It implies bowing with reverence. Together, "Ong Namo" means "I call on the infinite creative consciousness," and it opens you to the universal consciousness that guides all action.

"Guru" is the embodiment of the wisdom that one is seeking. "Dev" means higher, subtle, or divine. It refers to the spiritual realms. "Namo," at the end of the mantra, reaffirms the humble reverence of the student. Taken together, "Guru Dev Namo" means, "I call on the divine wisdom," whereby you bow before your higher self to guide you in using the knowledge and energy given by the cosmic self.

MENTAL FOCUS

Meditation requires concentration. To receive the benefits of each meditation, you will need to mentally focus. To assist you, the instructions for each meditation will tell you where to focus your concentration with your eyes. Unless you are directed to do otherwise, close your eyes and focus at the Third Eye Point. It is located between the eyebrows, where the root of the nose meets the skull bone.

Mentally locate this point by gently turning your eyes upward and inward. Remain aware of your breath, your posture, your hand position(s), your movements, and any mantra that may accompany the meditation. Be aware of it all as you center your awareness at the place of focus. This may sound like a lot at first. However, as with anything, the more you do it, the more it becomes second nature. Meditation is a process. Be patient with yourself.

BREATH WITH MANTRA

Mantra are repeated sounds that direct and focus the mind. They are words of power. Mantra enables you to easily keep up throughout challenging exercises or meditations. The simplest movements have depth when mantra is applied. The power of the mantra is maximized when it is linked with your breath cycle. For example, Sat Naam, which rhymes with "But Mom," is a common mantra that means "Truth is my identity." Mentally repeat "Sat" on the inhale and "Naam" on the exhale. This will allow you to screen your thoughts so that each is a positive one.

PACING YOURSELF
Kundalini Yoga exercises may involve rhythmic movement between two or more postures. Begin slowly, keeping a steady rhythm. Then increase gradually as the body allows, being careful not to strain. Be sure that the spine has become warm and flexible before attempting rapid movements. It is important to be aware of your body and responsible for its well-being.

CONCLUDING AN EXERCISE
Unless it says otherwise, an exercise ends by inhaling and suspending the breath for a short time, then exhaling and relaxing the posture. While the breath is being held, apply the Root Lock[2], contracting the muscles around the anal sphincter, the sex organs, and the Navel Point, while drawing the navel back towards the spine. This consolidates the effects of any exercise and circulates the energy to your higher centers. Suspend the breath just beyond a level of comfort. If you experience any discomfort, immediately release the lock and exhale.

ENDING A YOGA PRACTICE
To close up a yoga practice, sit up straight and put the palms together, with the thumbs pointing up and resting against the sternum. Inhale deeply and chant the mantra SAT NAAM three times ("Sat" lasts 7 seconds, "Naam" 1 second.) The mantra means "Truth is my name" or "my true identity." This mantra connects you with your soul and your destination.

In Kundalini yoga classes or when practicing alone, we sing a short song before chanting three long Sat Naam. The song is an inspiring prayer for the rest of your day. It says: "May the Long Time Sun Shine Upon You, All Love Surround You, And the Pure Light Within You Guide Your Way On."[3]

---

[2] The Root Lock is like a hydraulic lock at the base of the spine. It coordinates, stimulates, and balances the energies involved with the rectum, sex organs, and Navel Point (i.e., the lower three chakras).

[3] You can find a beautiful version of this chant on the internet or go to the Gurbani Media Center from Sikhnet at sikhnet.com/gurbani/

ADVANCED KUNDALINI YOGA KRIYAS FROM THE LATE '90s

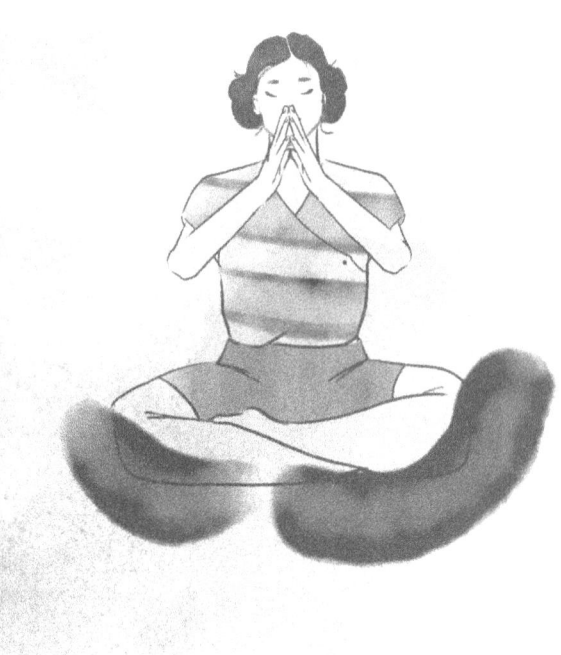

1 / Free Earthly Attachment and Give God a Chance

July 14, 1998

Sit in Easy Pose with a straight spine and a light Neck Lock.

Mudra: Touch the tips of the fingers to the corresponding fingers of the other hand, leaving space between the palms. Hold the mudra with the fingers pointing up and the tips of the Jupiter (index) fingers 6 inches (15 cm) in front of the nose, keeping the wrists straight. Press the fingertips together with equal pressure on each word of the mantra.

Eye Focus: Not specified.

Breath: Not specified.

Mantra: Chant the Guru Gaitri mantra with **4 HARs** for **10 minutes.** Then whistle with the music for **3 minutes.** (The recording by Nirinjan Kaur from *White Tantra Volume 1* was played in the original class.)

HAR HAR HAR HAR GOBINDAY
HAR HAR HAR HAR MUKUNDAY
HAR HAR HAR HAR UDAARAY
HAR HAR HAR HAR APAARAY
HAR HAR HAR HAR HAREEUNG
HAR HAR HAR HAR KAREEUNG
HAR HAR HAR HAR NIRNAAMAY
HAR HAR HAR HAR AKAAMAY

Total Time: 13 minutes.

To End: Inhale deeply, suspend the breath for **10 seconds**, look at yourself as a conscious being, and exhale completely with a whistle. Repeat **1 more time**. Inhale deeply, suspend the breath for **20 seconds**, press the fingertips together, consolidate your energy, and Cannon Fire exhale.

Comments: When we forget that we are made in God, we limit ourselves to earthly attachments. Ignoring the God within, attached to time, we dwell on the past, worry about the present, and fear the future, losing our limitless identity. Even at the time of death, we cling to our attachments, unable to release our subtle body to the One. When we focus on the infinite, we can experience God within our hearts and fearlessly enjoy each moment.

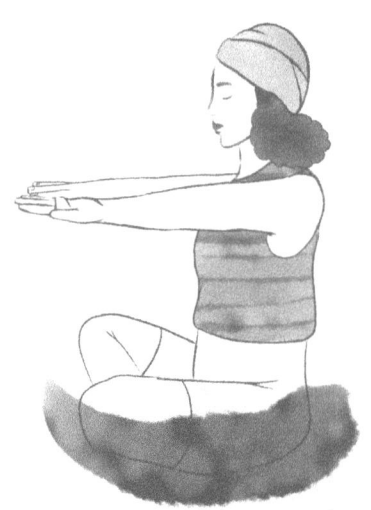

2 / Tuning Up the Frontal Lobe

August 3, 1998

Sit in Easy Pose with a straight spine and a light Neck Lock.

Mudra: Extend the arms straight forward, parallel to the ground and to each other. The right hand faces down, and the left hand faces up with the elbows straight.

Eye Focus: Not specified.

Breath: Breath of Fire.

Time: 11 minutes.

To End: Inhale deeply, suspend the breath for **15 seconds**, stretch out from the shoulders as far as possible and tighten the spine, and Cannon fire exhale. Repeat **2 more times**.

Comments: We are clever and live in a world where all information is at our fingertips, but we often lack commitment because we have not developed the frontal lobe. This kriya tunes up the frontal lobe, so we can realize the reality of our thoughts and avoid twisting them to hide ourselves or serve our egos, facing our desires, thoughts, and life situations straightforwardly.

breathe, rest, concentrate

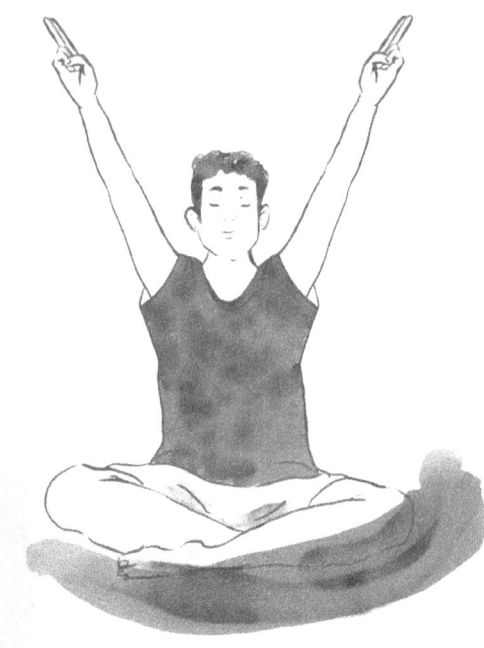

3 / **Meditation for Applied Consciousness**

August 25, 1998

Sit in Easy Pose with a straight spine and the head tilted slightly back.

Mudra: Extend the Jupiter (index) and Saturn (middle) fingers of both hands and hold the other fingers down with the thumbs. Stretch the arms out to the sides and up to 60 degrees, with no bend in the elbows or wrists and the palms facing up.

Eye Focus: Closed

Breath: Breath of Fire.

Time: 11 minutes.

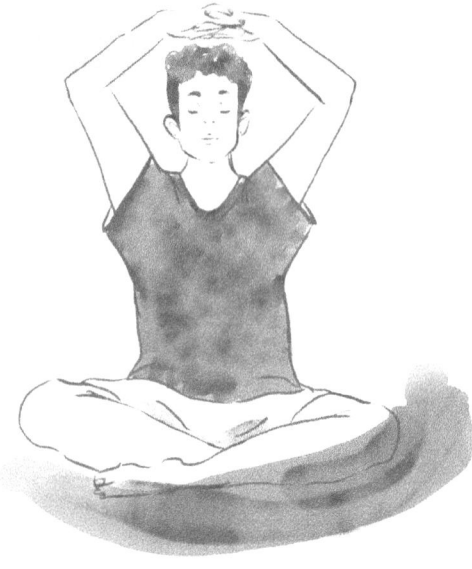

To End: Interlock the fingers in an arc a few inches above the head and pull the hands without separating them; continue Breath of Fire for **20 seconds.** Keeping the fingers interlaced, place them on the Navel Point, press the navel strongly, and continue Breath of Fire for another **30 seconds.** Inhale deeply, suspend the breath for **10 seconds**, press the hands on the Navel Point, squeeze the body, and exhale. Repeat **2 more times**, and Cannon Fire exhale the last time.

Comments: Focus on Infinity, not spirituality or religious ritual, and apply that perspective in everyday life. Facing life and acting from our higher Self is called applied consciousness. When our focus is on the divine, our circumstances will automatically change.

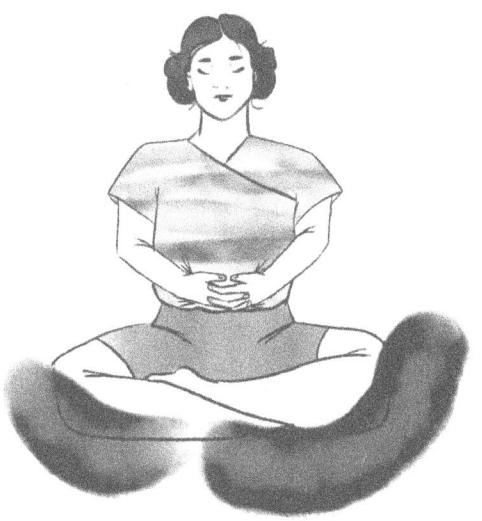

4 / Meditation for Inner Strength and Balance

August 31, 1998

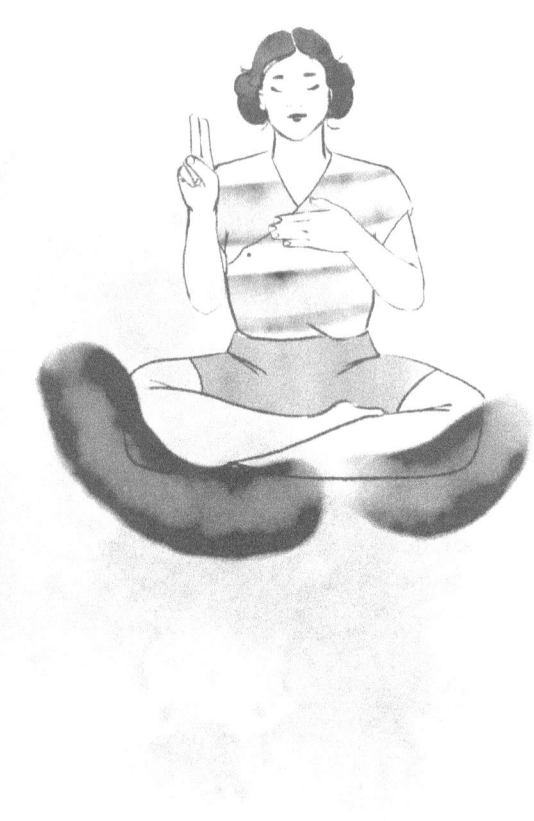

PART ONE
Sit in Easy Pose with a straight spine and a light Neck Lock.

Mudra: Bring the right hand by the shoulder with the palm facing forward. Extend the Jupiter (index) and Saturn (middle) fingers, and hold the other fingers down with the thumb. Place the left hand on the Heart Center with the fingers pointing to the right, thumb relaxed apart.

Eye Focus: Closed.

Breath and Mental Focus: Long Deep Breathing. Feel that you are pure, and that purity is breathing within you.

Time: 3-5 minutes. Immediately begin Part Two.

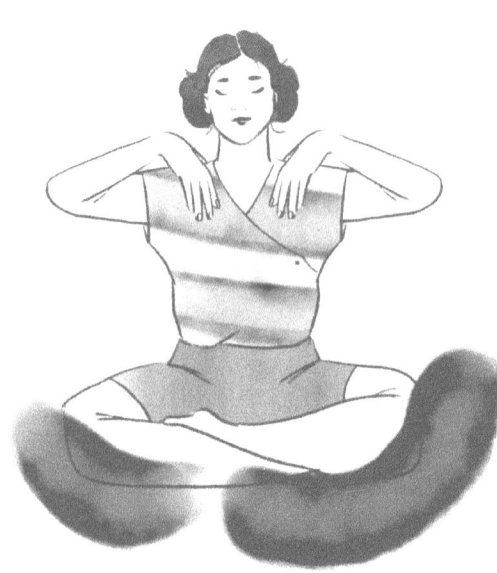

PART TWO
Remain in Easy Pose.

Mudra: Place the hands on the shoulders, with the elbows out to the sides and the upper arms parallel to the ground.

Eye Focus: Not specified.

Breath: Long Deep Breathing.

Time: 3-5 minutes. Immediately begin Part Three.

Comments: This exercise builds inner strength to bear the weight of life

PART THREE

Remain in Easy Pose.

Mudra: Extend the arms out to the sides parallel to the ground with the palms facing up, fingers together, and thumbs relaxed.

Eye Focus: Not specified.

Breath: Long Deep Breathing.

Time: 3-5 minutes.

To End: Inhale deeply, suspend the breath for **15 seconds**, exhale.

Comments: This meditation is to be practiced for 11 consecutive days for the same amount of time, rest for 7 days, then practice again for 11 days, rest for 7 days, and then practice for 11 more days. The minimum time is 3 minutes for each exercise (total of 9 minutes) and 2 minutes for relaxation. We can be successful in life through luck, hard work, or with someone's assistance. And there is a fourth way: when the mind is balanced. Yogis say that breathing is the quickest way to affect the mind. We can develop steadiness of mind when we daily practice Long Deep Breathing and conscious yogic breathing.

5 / Expand to Create Momentum

September 9, 1998

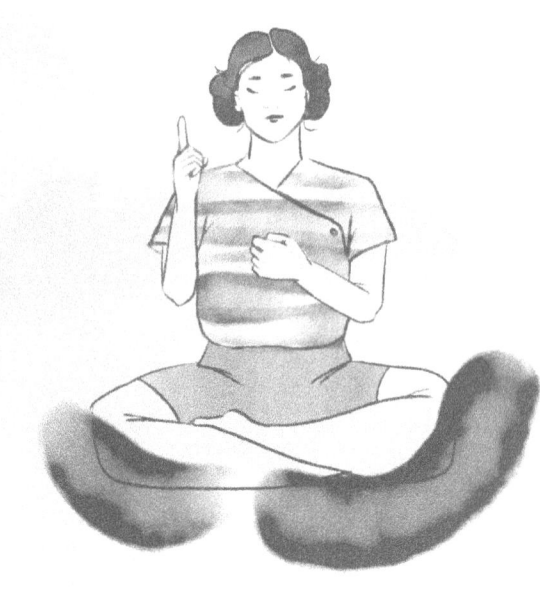

AYKAA MAA-EE JUGAT VI-AA-EE TIN CHAYLAY PARVAAN.
IK SANSAAREE IK BHANDAAREE IK LAA-AY DEEBAAN.
JIV TIS BHAAVAI TIVAI CHALAAVAI JIV HOVAI FURMAAN.
OH VAYKHAI ONAA NADAR NA AAVAI BAHUTAA AYHU VIDAAN.
AADAYS TISAI AADAYS.
AAD ANEEL ANAAD ANAAHAT JUG JUG AYKO VAYS.

PART ONE
Sit in Easy Pose with a straight spine and a light Neck Lock.

Mudra: Make a fist of the left hand and place it on the Heart Center. Extend the right Jupiter (index) finger and hold the other fingers down with the thumb. Place the right hand in front of the body with the wrist at the level of the shoulder, the forearm perpendicular to the ground, and the palm facing left.

Eye Focus: Closed.

Breath: Not specified.

Mantra: Chant the 30th Pauree of Japji Sahib. (Live music was played in the original class.)

Time: 24 minutes.

To End: Inhale deeply, exhale, and begin Part Two.

PART TWO
Remain in Easy Pose.

Mudra: Grasp the opposite elbows with the hands and raise the forearms up to shoulder level, parallel to the ground.

Eye Focus: Not specified.

Breath: Not specified.

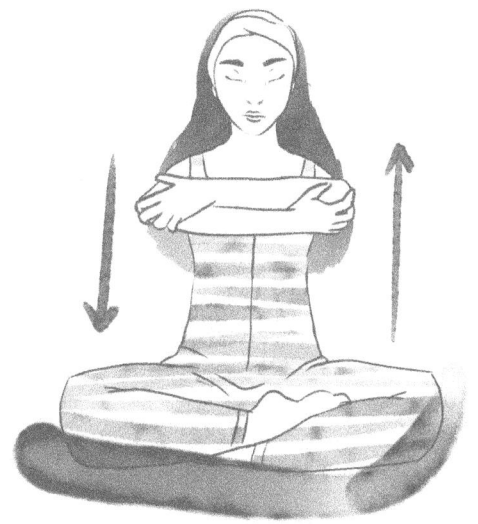

Mantra:
a) Continue to chant the 30th Pauree of Japji Sahib for **4 minutes**.
b) Chant **HAR** from the navel once per second for **2 ½ minutes**. ("Rhythms of Gatka" by Mata Mandir Singh was played in the original class.)
c) Chant **HAR** from the navel and move the forearms up and down **6 inches** (15 cm) from the starting position in rhythm with the chanting for **2 minutes**. ("Rhythms of Gatka" by Mata Mandir Singh was played in the original class.)

Total Time: 8 ½ minutes.

To End: Inhale, exhale, and relax.

CONTINUE ON NEXT PAGE »

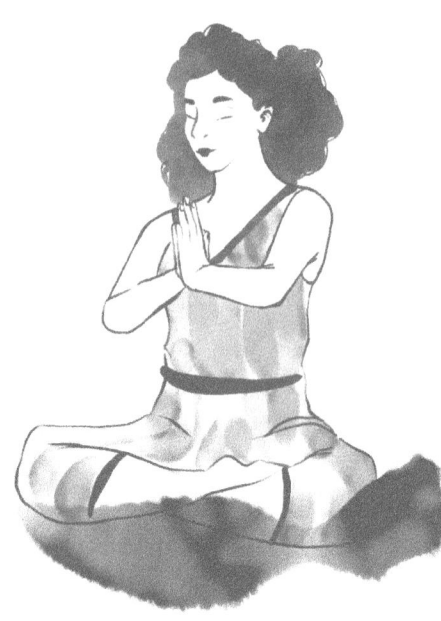

PART THREE
Remain in Easy Pose.

Mudra: Place the hands in Prayer Pose, creating an angle of 10 degrees from the elbows to the wrists. The hands are about 12 inches (30 cm) in front of the chest.

Eye Focus: Not specified.

Breath: Not specified.

Mantra: Chant the 30th Pauree of Japji Sahib from the Navel.

Time: 2 minutes.

To End: Inhale, exhale, and begin Part Four.

PART FOUR
Remain in Easy Pose.

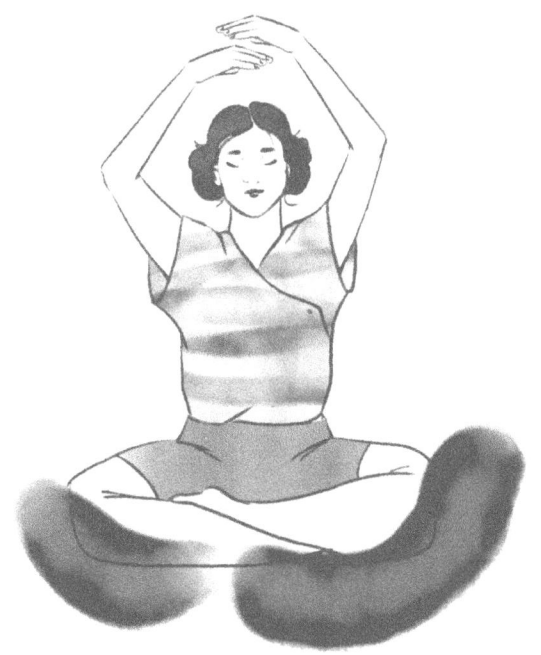

Mudra: Bring the arms in an arc over the head, the left hand 4 inches (10 cm) above the right, with palms facing down.

Eye Focus: Not specified.

Breath: Not specified.

Mantra: Chant **RAKHAY RAKHANHAAR.** (The recording by Singh Kaur was played in the original class.)

**RAKHAY RAKHANHAAR AAP UBAARIUN
GUR KEE PAIREE PAA-EH KAAJ SAVAARIUN
HOAA AAP DAYAAL MANHO NA VISAARIUN
SAADH JANAA KAI SUNG BHAVJAL TAARIUN
SAAKAT NINDAK DUSHT KHIN MAA-EH BIDAARIUN
TIS SAAHIB KEE TAYK NAANAK MANAI MAA-EH
JIS SIMRAT SUKH HO-EH SAGLAY DOOKH JAA-EH**

Time: 2 minutes.

To End: Inhale, exhale, and begin Part Five.

CONTINUE ON NEXT PAGE »

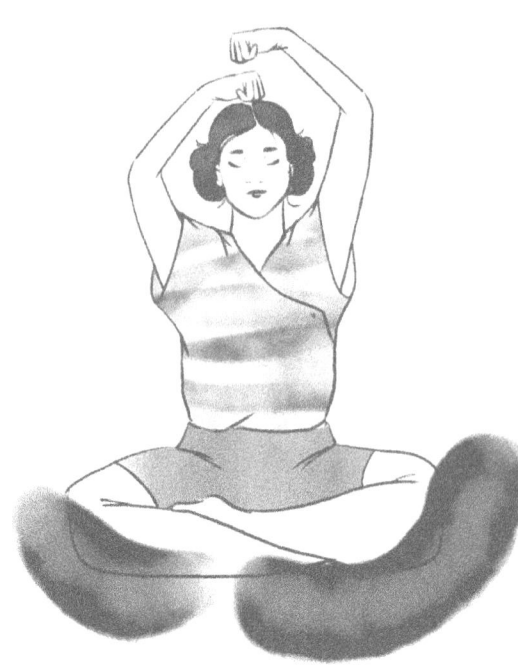

PART FIVE
Remain in Easy Pose.

Mudra: Maintain the same posture as Part Four, and make the hands into fists.

Eye Focus: Not specified.

Breath: Not specified.

Mantra: Chant the mantra **KAAL AKAAL.** (The recording by Guru Shabad Singh Khalsa was played in the original class.)

**KAAL AKAAL SIREE AKAAL
MAHAA AKAAL
AKAAL MOORAT WHAA-HAY GUROO**

Time: 2 minutes.

To End: Inhale, exhale, and begin Part Six.

PART SIX
Remain in Easy Pose.

Mudra: Interlace the fingers and stretch the arms up straight above the head.

Eye Focus: Not specified.

Breath: Not specified.

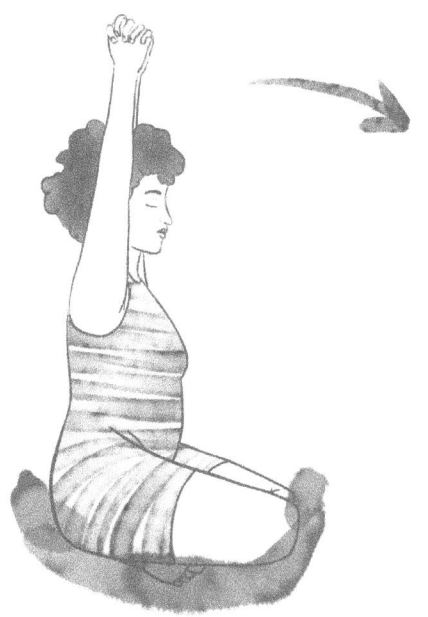
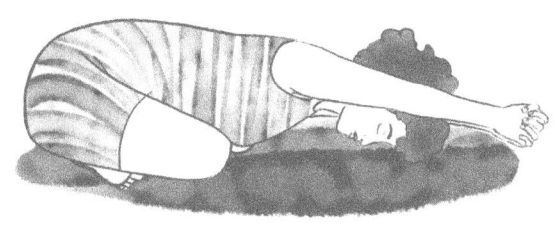

Mantra:

a) Chant the mantra **SAT NAAM WHAA-HAY GUROO** from the navel. Bend forward, bring the hands and forehead to the ground on **SAT NAAM** and come up on **WHAA-HAY GUROO** for the first **1 minute**. (The recording by Lata Mangeshkar was played in the original class.)

b) Listen to a musical recording of Jaap Sahib, sit meditatively for the first stanza, and bring the hands and forehead to the ground every time you hear "Namastang" or "Namo" for **4 ½ minutes**. Without the recording, the movement is done to 10 beats as follows: Bow down and come up in 2 counts for 4 cycles, and rest in the starting position on counts 9 and 10. (The recording "Jaap Sahib" by Satnam Singh Sethi was played in the original class.)

Time: 5 ½ minutes.

To End: Inhale deeply, exhale, and relax.

Comments: Your consciousness naturally expands when you meditate on Infinity. That state creates a vacuum, which Mother Nature replenishes. Refusing to be limited results in strong momentum toward prosperity and fulfillment.

6 / Meditation in Action

September 10, 1998

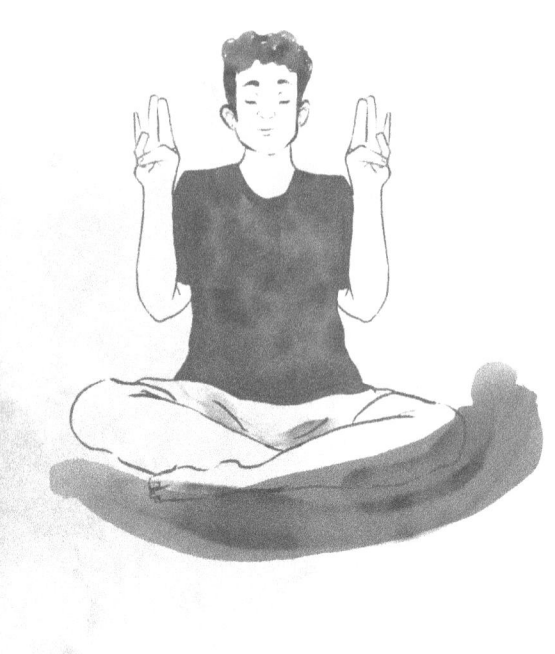

PART ONE
Sit in Easy Pose with a straight spine and a light Neck Lock.

Mudra: Touch the tips of the thumbs and Sun (ring) fingers together, and extend the other fingers straight up in Ravi Mudra. Bring the hands by the shoulders with the elbows relaxed at the sides and the palms facing forward.

Eye Focus: Not specified.

Breath: Not specified.

Mantra: Chant **CHATTR CHAKKR VARTEE** from the navel. (The recording by Kulwant Singh was played in the original class.)

Time: 28 minutes.

To End: Inhale, exhale, and immediately begin Part Two.

**CHATTR CHAKKR VARTEE,
CHATTR CHAKKR
BHUGATAY
SUYUMBHAV SUBHANG
SARAB DAA SARAB JUGTAY
DUKAALANG PRANAASEE
DAYAALANG SAROOPAY
SADAA UNG SUNGAY
ABHANGANG BIBHOOTAY**

PART TWO
Remain in Easy Pose.

Mudra: Maintain the hands at shoulder level and bend the wrists so the palms are facing up, parallel to the ground, with fingers together and pointing out to the sides. Keep the fingers straight and the palm flat.

Eye Focus: Not specified.

Breath: Not specified.

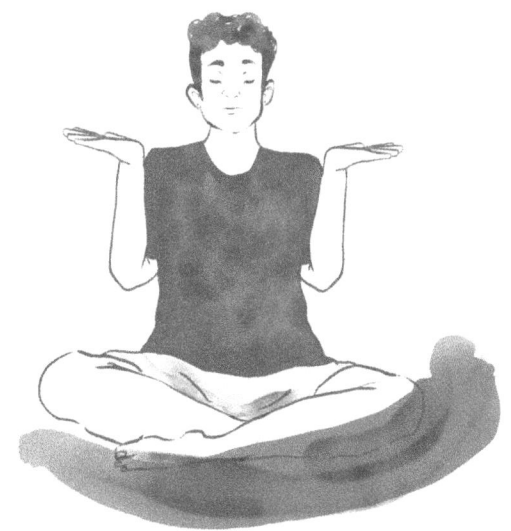

Mantra:
a) Continue chanting **CHATTR CHAKKR VARTEE** for **3 minutes**.
b) Become thoughtless and sit in silence for **2 ½ minutes**.
c) Chant **HUMEE HUM BRAHM HUM** from the navel for **4 minutes**. (The recording by Nirinjan Kaur was played in the original class.)

Total Time: 9 ½ minutes.

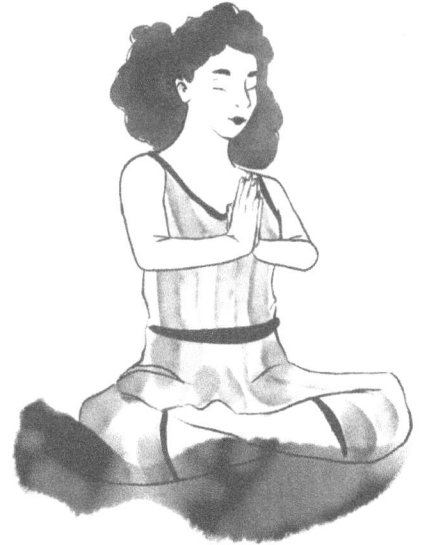

To End: Inhale deeply and bring the hands into Prayer Pose at the Heart Center, pressing the palms together strongly and squeezing the whole body. Suspend the breath for **10 seconds**, and exhale. Repeat **2 more times**. Shake out the hands for a few seconds.

Comments: Questioning yourself creates duality, and acting from duality creates karma, or consequences. When you act from a meditative mind, there is no question; thus, what you do creates no karma. This is dharmic living, as an integrated being in action.

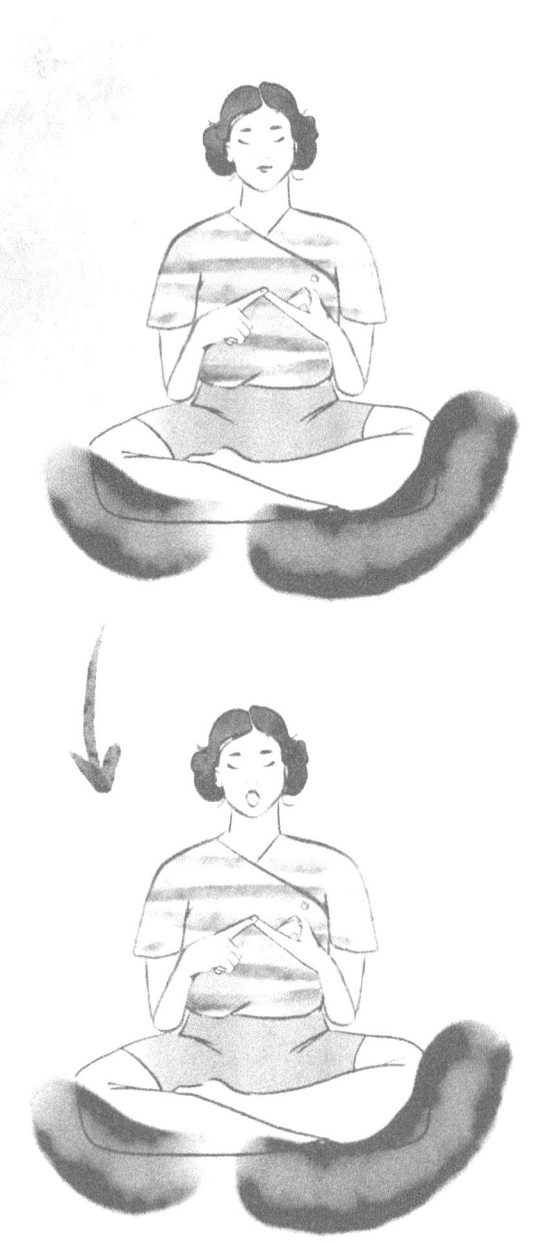

7 / Shine Your Light

September 23, 1998

PART ONE
Sit in Easy Pose with a straight spine and a light Neck Lock.

Mudra: Rest the elbows against the body. Extend the Jupiter (index) fingers of both hands and hold the other fingers down with the thumbs. Place the pad of the right Jupiter (index) finger on the pad of the left Jupiter finger, right palm facing down, left palm facing up. Hold the mudra pointing forward with the forearms parallel to the ground.

Eye Focus: 1/10th open.

Breath:
a) Inhale deeply through the mouth with a whistle; exhale in a stroke through the nose. Continue for **20 minutes**.
b) Inhale deeply through the "O" mouth, suspend the breath for as long as possible, and exhale through the nose. Make the breath as long as possible. Continue for **1 ½ minutes**.

Mental Focus: Make your body like a candle and radiate your spirit.

Total Time: 21 ½ minutes.
Immediately begin Part Two.

PART TWO
Remain in Easy Pose.

Mudra: Place the palms together with the first section of the fingers alternating and lined up next to each other; the right Jupiter finger (index), the left Jupiter finger, the right Saturn (middle) finger, the left Saturn, and so on, with the left Mercury (little) finger last. Stretch the arms straight forward from the shoulders, parallel to the ground, pointing forward.

Eye Focus: Looking at the hands through closed eyes.

Breath: Long Deep Breathing.

Time: 1 ½ minutes.

To End: Inhale deeply, suspend the breath for **10-15 seconds**, stretch the arms more, squeeze the body, and exhale. Repeat **2 more times**.

Comments: Spirituality is three-fold: our bodies are known to us, our minds are controlled by us, and our spirits radiate from us. We are just like candles; we have wax, we have wicks inside, but if it is not lit, it doesn't emit light. When we are radiant, the universe provides for us.

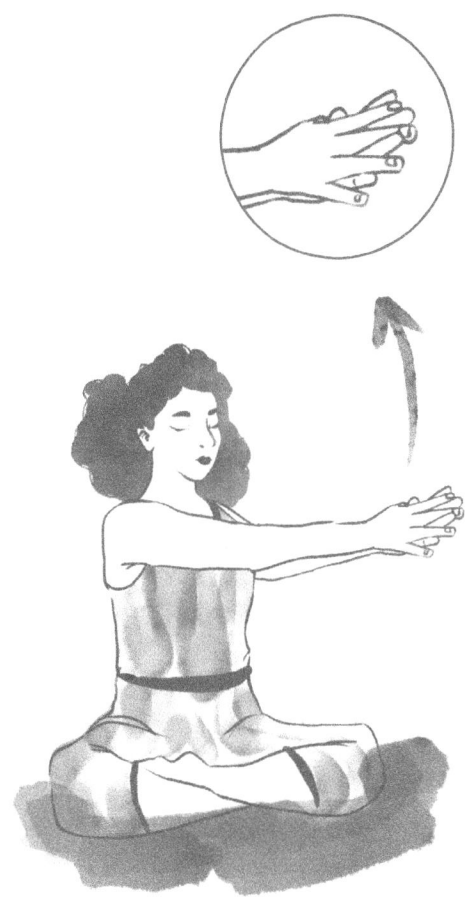

BE YOU

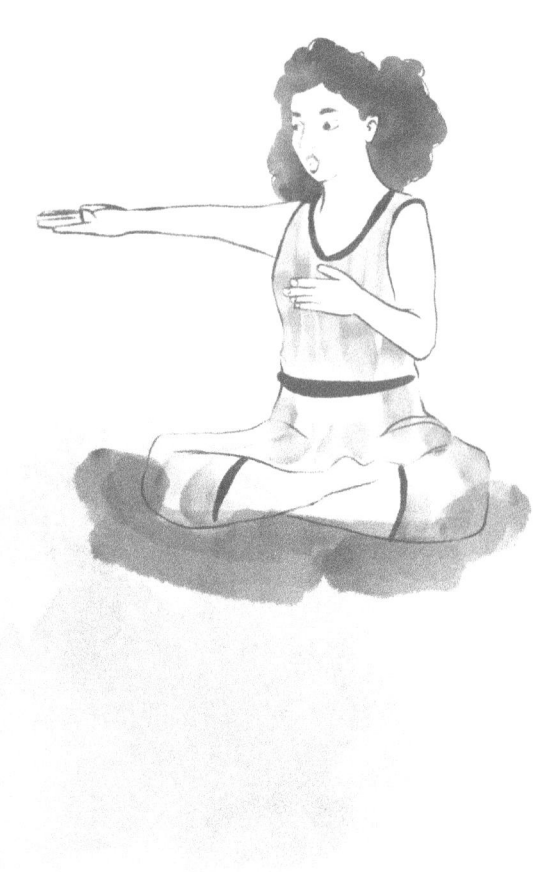

8 / Meditation to Become Divine

September 24, 1998

Sit in Easy Pose with a straight spine and a light Neck Lock.

Mudra: Place the left hand on the Heart Center with the fingers pointing to the right. Stretch the right arm straight forward, parallel to the ground, with no bend in the wrist or elbow, with the right hand facing up, fingers together, and thumb relaxed.

Eye Focus: Look at the right hand.

Breath: Inhale deeply through the nose and exhale strongly through the "O" mouth so that the breath is felt on the right palm.

Time: 18 minutes.

To End: Inhale deeply, exhale powerfully, and suspend the breath out for **5-10 seconds**. Quickly inhale, exhale twice, and suspend the breath out for **5-10 seconds**. Inhale, exhale, suspend the breath out and squeeze the body for **5-10 seconds**.

Comments: If we know ourselves, know our surroundings, and know our worth, we can live content and self-contained. This is the way to settle our karmas and live divinely in this world.

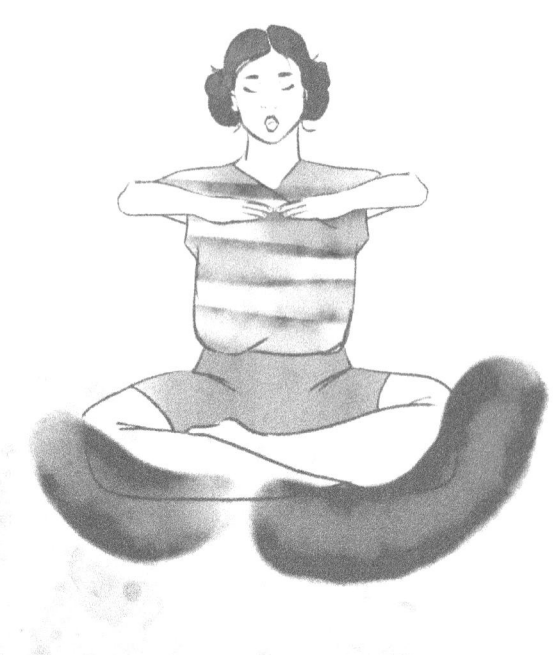

9 / **Raise Your Vibration to Heal Others**

September 28, 1998

Sit in Easy Pose with a straight spine and a light Neck Lock.

Mudra: Stretch the arms forward at shoulder level parallel to the ground, elbows slightly bent to create a circle in front of the body, with palms facing down and a gap between the fingers.

Eye Focus: Tip of the Nose.

Breath: Not specified.

Mantra:
a) Chant **SAT NAAM WHAA-HAY GUROO** from the navel. Continue for **11 minutes**. (The recording by Lata Mangeshkar was played in the original class.)
b) Chant **HAR** and pull the navel strongly with each repetition. Continue for **5 ½ minutes**. ("Rhythms of Gatka" by Mata Mandir Singh was played in the original class.)
c) Do Breath of Fire in rhythm with the drums. Continue for **4 ½ minutes**. Inhale deeply, suspend the breath, and Cannon Fire

exhale. ("Rhythms of Gatka" by Mata Mandir Singh was played in the original class.)

d) Chant **ARDAAS BHAEE**. Continue for **3 ½ minutes**. (The instrumental version of Ardas Bhaee from the album *Healing Sounds of the Ancients #5* was played in the original class.)

**ARDAAS BHAEE, AMAR DAAS GUROO,
AMAR DAAS GUROO, ARDAAS BHAEE,
RAAM DAAS GUROO, RAAM DAAS GUROO,
RAAM DAAS GUROO, SUCHEE SAHEE**

Total Time: 23 ½ minutes.

To End: Inhale deeply, suspend the breath for **15 seconds**, squeeze the whole body, and Cannon Fire exhale. Repeat **1 more time**.

Comments: Start with 3 minutes per part, and slowly build up to 11 minutes per part. Our electromagnetic field and psyche create our biorhythms. Sometimes we confuse these rhythms for who we really are. Raising our vibration with this practice increases our healing light.

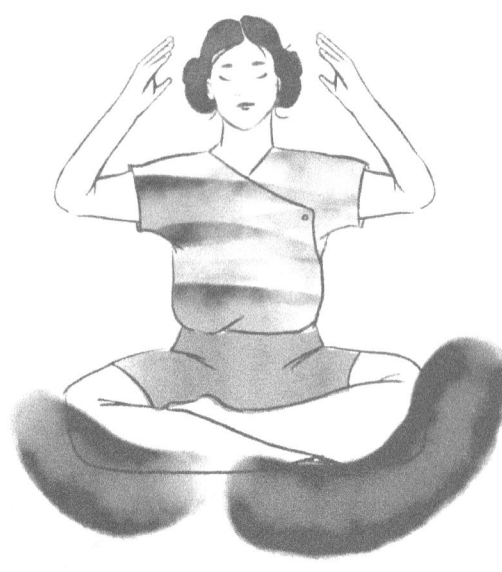

10 / **See With An Infinite Perspective**

September 29, 1998

PART ONE
Sit in Easy Pose with a straight spine and a light Neck Lock.

Mudra: Bring the hands up 6 inches (15 cm) to the sides of the ears. Palms are slightly cupped facing the head, with the thumbs stretched towards the ears.

Eye Focus: Tip of the Nose.

Breath: Long Deep Breathing.

Time: 25 ½ minutes. Immediately begin Part Two.

PART TWO
Remain in Easy Pose.

Mudra: Place the hands on the Heart Center, right over left.

Eye Focus: Closed.

Breath: Not specified.

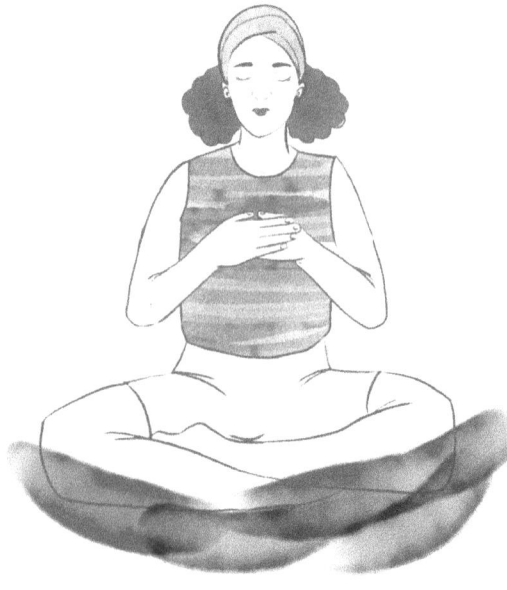

Mantra: Whistle with the music. (The instrumental version of Ardas Bhaee from the album *Healing Sounds of the Ancients #5* was played in the original class.)

Time: 2 minutes.

To End: Inhale deeply, suspend the breath for **10 seconds**, press the hands firmly on the Heart Center, and Cannon Fire exhale. Repeat **2 more times**.

Comments: When we see through the Third Eye, instead of the personal "I," we remember our relationship with infinity. We see circumstances from a broader perspective. From this vantage point, we view our value, our light, and our essence, and we can forgive ourselves. Our awareness expands, and we understand that all things come from the Divine.

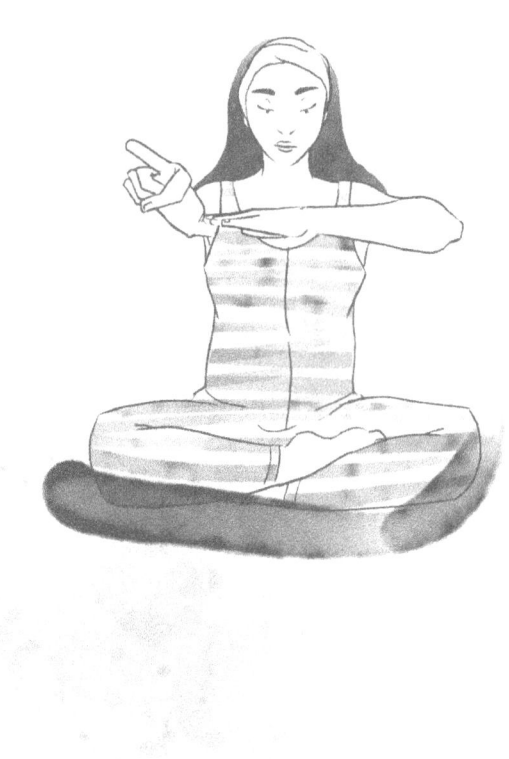

11 / **Become Sensitive and Alert**

October 5, 1998

PART ONE
Sit in Easy Pose with a straight spine and a light Neck Lock.

Mudra: Extend the right Jupiter (index) finger and hold the other fingers down with the thumb. Stretch the right arm straight forward, parallel to the ground, with the palm facing down. With the left Saturn (middle) finger, touch the crease inside the right elbow and keep the left arm parallel to the ground with the palm facing down. The fingers of the left hand are straight.

Eye Focus: Tip of the Nose.

Breath: Breath of Fire.

Time: 2 ½ minutes.

To End: Inhale, exhale, and begin Part Two.

PART TWO
Remain in Easy Pose.

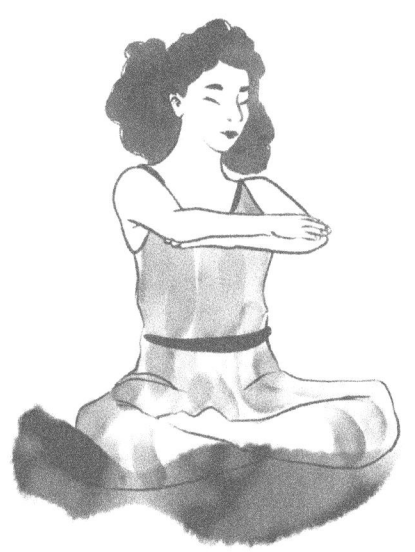

Mudra: Keep the left hand in the same position as Part One, and place the right forearm on top of the left forearm at shoulder level.

Eye Focus: Not specified.

Mantra and Breath:
a) Breath of Fire for **2 minutes**.
b) Chant **WHAA-HAY GUROO, WHAA-HAY GUROO, WHAA-HAY GUROO, WHAA-HAY JEEO** from the navel with the tip of the tongue for **4 ½ minutes**. (The recording by Giani Ji was played in the original class.)
c) Chant **HAR** from the navel in rhythm with the drums for **4 ½ minutes**. (The recording "Rhythms of Gatka" by Mata Mandir Singh was played in the original class.)

Total Time: 11 minutes.

To End: Inhale and suspend the breath briefly. Exhale and begin Part Three.

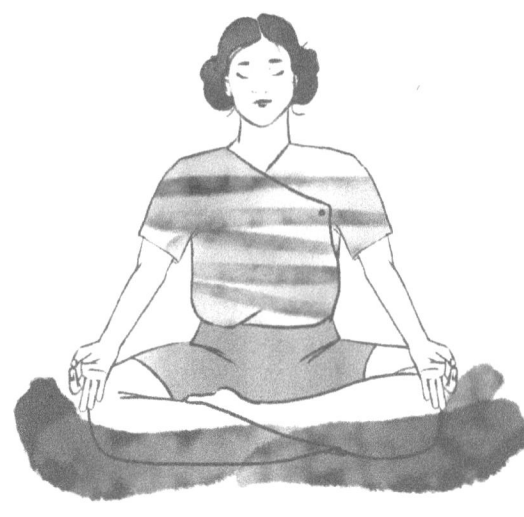

PART THREE
Remain in Easy Pose.

Mudra: Place the wrists on the knees and touch the tips of the thumbs and the Jupiter (index) fingers together in Gyan Mudra. Keep the arms straight.

Eye Focus: Not specified.

Breath: Not specified.

Mantra: Chant the Guru Gaitri mantra with **4 HARs**. (The recording "Har Har Har Har Gobinde" by Nirinjan Kaur, from *White Tantra Volume 1*, was played in the original class.)

**HAR HAR HAR HAR GOBINDAY
HAR HAR HAR HAR MUKUNDAY
HAR HAR HAR HAR UDAARAY
HAR HAR HAR HAR APAARAY
HAR HAR HAR HAR HAREEUNG
HAR HAR HAR HAR KAREEUNG
HAR HAR HAR HAR NIRNAAMAY
HAR HAR HAR HAR AKAAMAY**

Time: 4 ½ minutes.

To End: Inhale, exhale, and immediately begin Part Four.

PART FOUR
Remain in the posture.

Eye Focus: Not specified.

Breath: Not specified.

Mantra: Chant **RAKHAY RAKHANHAAR**. (The recording by Singh Kaur was played in the original class.)

**RAKHAY RAKHANHAAR AAP UBAARIUN
GUR KEE PAIREE PAA-EH KAAJ SAVAARIUN
HOAA AAP DAYAAL MANHO NA VISAARIUN
SAADH JANAA KAI SUNG BHAVJAL TAARIUN
SAAKAT NINDAK DUSHT KHIN MAA-EH BIDAARIUN
TIS SAAHIB KEE TAYK NAANAK MANAI MAA-EH
JIS SIMRAT SUKH HO-EH SAGLAY DOOKH JAA-EH**

Time: 3 minutes.

To End: Inhale deeply, suspend the breath for **5-10 seconds**, and Cannon Fire exhale. Repeat **2 more times**.

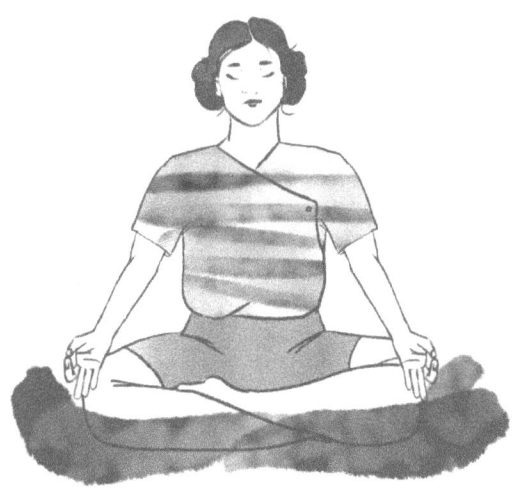

Comments: The mind makes decisions in a fraction of a second that have consequences and, over time, create our patterns of reacting. When the mind fails to record circumstances accurately, it triggers an incorrect response, either in our words or actions. Communication is a relay of a frequency; it is effective when the frequencies of the sender and the receiver match. To avoid painful feelings, we can become numb, and this keeps us from being able to tune into others' frequencies. We may not be aware of our pattern of denying our emotions until later in life. Instead, we can forgive ourselves and others for what happened in the past, relate to our psyches deeply, and meet the energy of others authentically. This kriya helps us become sensitive and alert, so reality penetrates our minds and we respond effectively and intelligently.

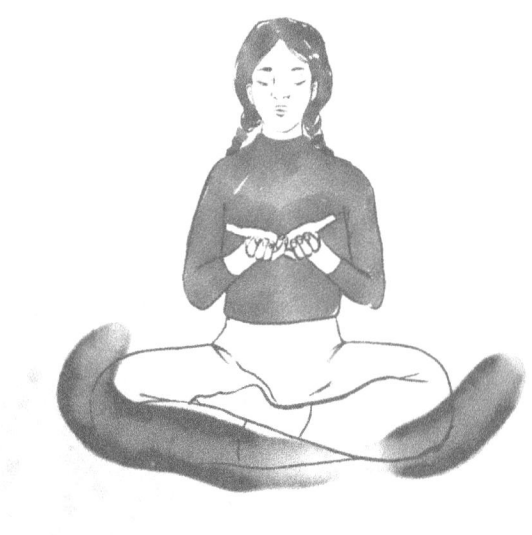

12 / **Make Progress in Life**

October 8, 1998

Sit in Easy Pose with a straight spine and a light Neck Lock.

Mudra: Bring the hands together at the level of the center of the chest, hands facing up, slightly cupped, elbows and upper arms relaxed. Hook the Mercury (little) fingers and keep the other fingers together with thumbs separated.

Eye Focus: Tip of the Nose.

Breath: Breath of Fire.

Time: 22 ½ minutes.

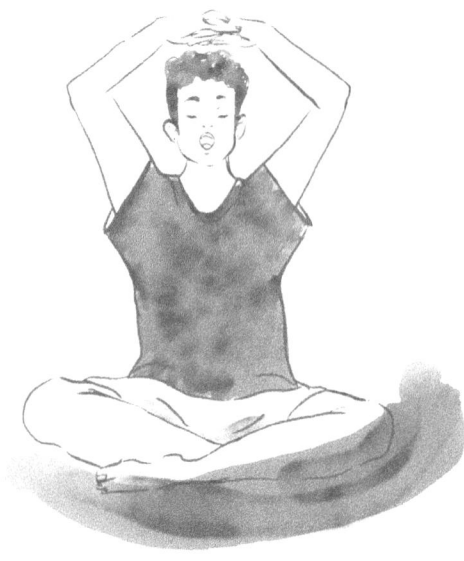

To End: Hold the posture and begin Breath of Fire through the mouth for **45 seconds**. Interlace the hands in an arc over the head and continue Breath of Fire through the mouth for **45 seconds**. Inhale deeply, suspend the breath, stretch the spine up for **5-10 seconds**, and Cannon Fire exhale. Repeat this breath 2 more times. Relax. ("Pantra" and "Rhythms of Gatka" by Matamandir Singh were played in the original class. Gong was played over the recording in the last few minutes of the exercise.)

Comments: Life can become like a treadmill; we walk for an hour and remain in the same place. In this kriya, praana and apana activate the *udhana vayu*[4] to help us get off this treadmill and actually progress.

---

[4] Udhana vauy is one of the five primary vayus, which are different frequencies and modes of motion of the Prana. It resides in the larynx and upwards into the head. As opposed to prana, it throws the air up and out. It is about projection. It is active in all forms of speech as well as in expelling through vomiting. It interacts with all the senses in the head. When udhana is not properly regulated, the voice can be irregular. If udhana is strong, you can project, and you can create with your word.

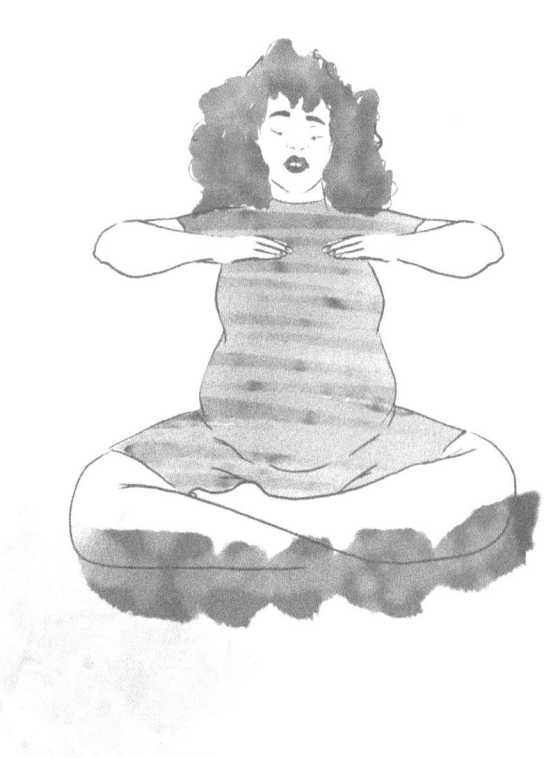

13 / Creative Thought and Action for Success

October 9, 1998

Sit in Easy Pose with a straight spine and a light Neck Lock.

Mudra: Bring the forearms parallel to the ground, with elbows to the sides and the hands in front of the chest. The palms face down with the fingers pointing towards each other with a gap between them. The fingers are together and straight, thumbs stretched towards the body.

Eye Focus: Tip of the Nose.

Breath & Mantra:
a) Chant **HAR** from the navel for **18 ½ minutes**. ("Rhythms of Gatka" by Matamandir Singh was played in the original class).
b) Do Breath of Fire for **1 ½ minutes**.
c) Chant the mantra **RAKHAY RAKHANHAAR** for **2 minutes**. (The recording by Singh Kaur was played in the original class).
d) Whistle with the music for **1 minute**.

RAKHAY RAKHANHAAR AAP UBAARIUN
GUR KEE PAIREE PAA-EH KAAJ SAVAARIUN
HOAA AAP DAYAAL MANHO NA VISAARIUN
SAADH JANAA KAI SUNG BHAVJAL TAARIUN
SAAKAT NINDAK DUSHT KHIN MAA-EH BIDAARIUN
TIS SAAHIB KEE TAYK NAANAK MANAI MAA-EH
JIS SIMRAT SUKH HO-EH SAGLAY DOOKH JAA-EH

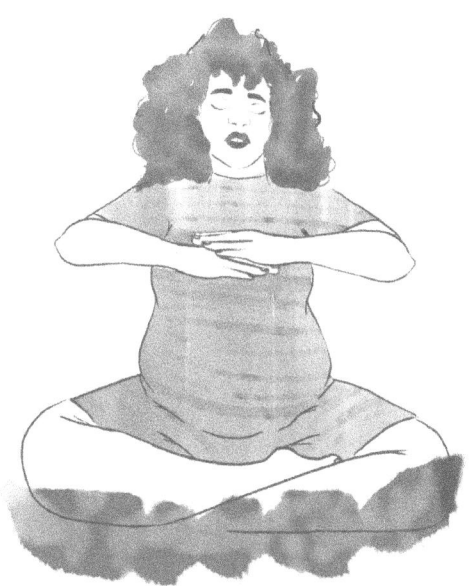

Total Time: 23 minutes.

To End: Hold the posture, inhale deeply, suspend the breath for **15 seconds**, tighten the body, then exhale. Inhale deeply, placing the right hand on top of the left, keeping the arms parallel to the ground. Suspend the breath for **15 seconds** and tighten the body, then exhale. Inhale deeply, interlace the hands, stretch the arms up straight, suspend the breath for **15 seconds**, tighten the body, and then exhale.

Comments: In this mudra, the gap between the fingers represents the gap between thoughts. When the psyche fills this gap with creative thought, how we choose to act is automatically positive. Actions based on a creative thought protect us from negative vibrations. This is a fundamental human strength that allows us to confront any situation and achieve success.

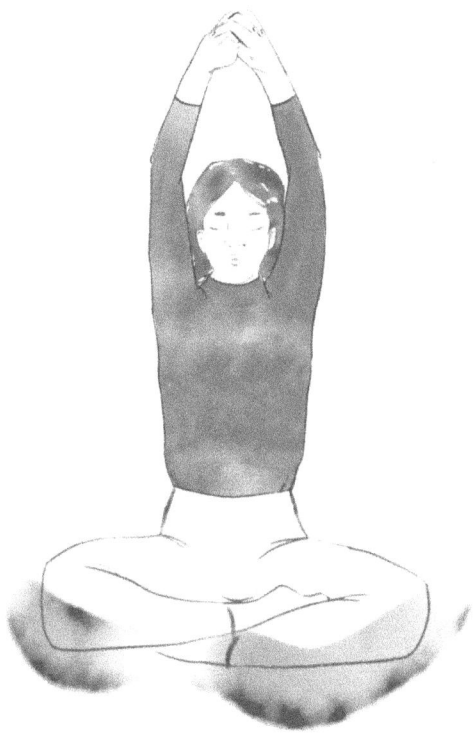

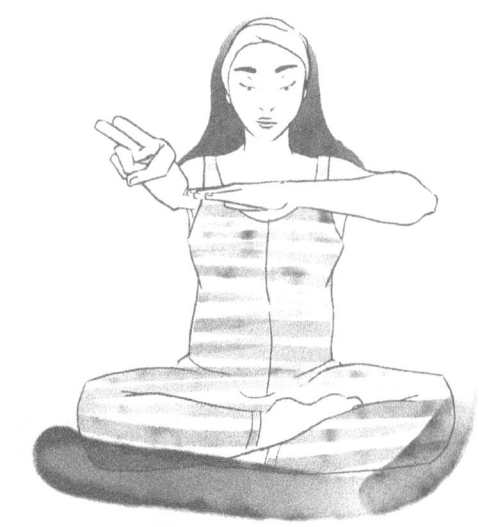

14 / Access Reserve Strength to Confront Reality

October 17, 1998

PART ONE
Sit in Easy Pose with a straight spine and a light Neck Lock.

Mudra: Extend the Jupiter (index) and Saturn (middle) fingers with the other fingers held down by the thumb. Stretch the right arm forward, parallel to the ground, with no bend in the elbow, palm facing down. Place the left hand at the level of the Heart Center, forearm parallel to the ground, palm facing down, and fingers pointing towards the right. Touch the tip of the left Saturn (middle) finger to the vein in the crease on the inside of the right elbow.

Eye Focus: Tip of the Nose.

Breath: Long Deep Breathing with a brief suspension after the inhalation.

Time: 11 minutes.

To End: Inhale deeply, squeeze

the body, stretch the arms up, and lengthen the spine; suspend the breath for **10 seconds**, and exhale. Inhale deeply, stretch the arms and the spine, and distribute the energy through every cell of the body. Suspend the breath for **15 seconds**, and Cannon Fire exhale. Repeat the breath **1 more time**.

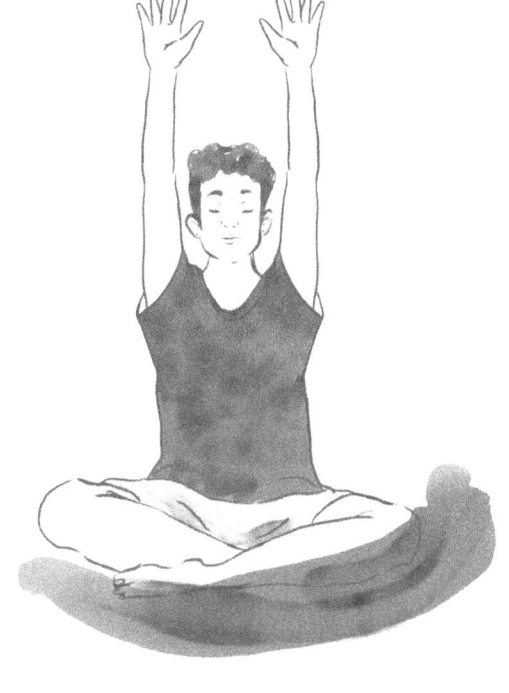

PART TWO
Remain in Easy Pose with a straight spine and a light Neck Lock.

Mudra: Press the palms firmly over the ears, with the elbows out to the sides, the fingers together pointing backward, and the thumbs separated from the hand.

Eye Focus: Not specified.

Breath: Not specified.

Mantra: Chant **HAR** from the navel at a pace of one repetition per second. Listen to the sounds you are making as you chant. (The recording "Pantra" by Mata Mandir Singh was played in the original class.)

Time: 5 minutes.

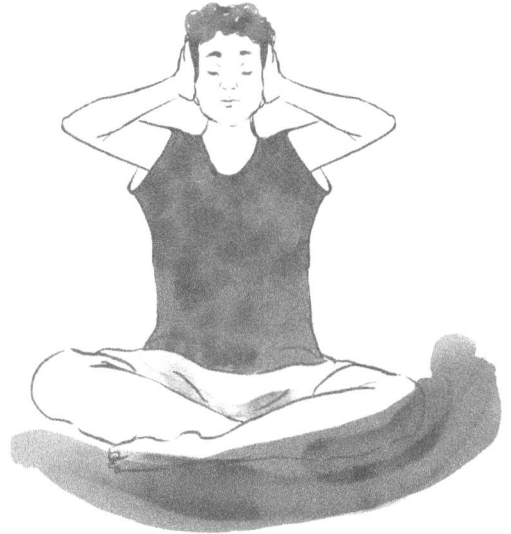

CONTINUE ON NEXT PAGE »

To End: Inhale deeply, suspend the breath for **10 seconds**, press the ears with the hands, tighten the whole body, and Cannon Fire exhale.

Comment: This exercise moves energy through the *Sushumna*, the central nervous system.

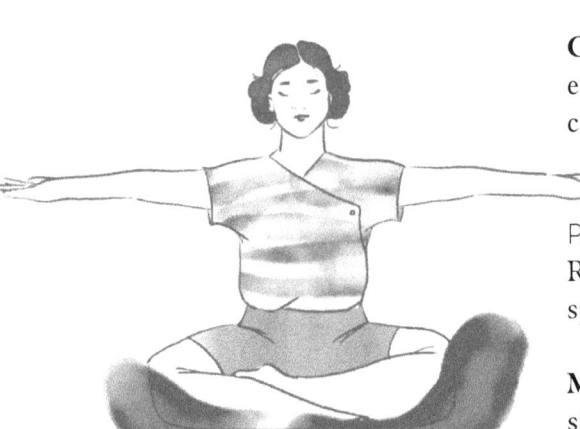

PART THREE

Remain in Easy Pose with a straight spine and a light Neck Lock.

Mudra: Extend the arms out to the sides at shoulder level, parallel to the ground with no bend in the elbows, palms facing up with fingers together and tensed, and the thumbs stretched away, pointing behind. Firmly twist the arms backward and keep the posture steady.

Eye Focus: Not specified.

Breath: Not specified.

Mantra: Whistle with the music. (The instrumental version of Ardas Bhaee from the album *Healing Sounds of the Ancients #5* was played in the original class.)

Time: 4 minutes.

To End: Inhale deeply, exhale, and immediately begin Part Four.

Comments: Twist the elbows more to help release pain and tension. This exercise may alleviate both conscious and subconscious anxiety.

PART FOUR
Remain in Easy Pose with a straight spine and a light Neck Lock.

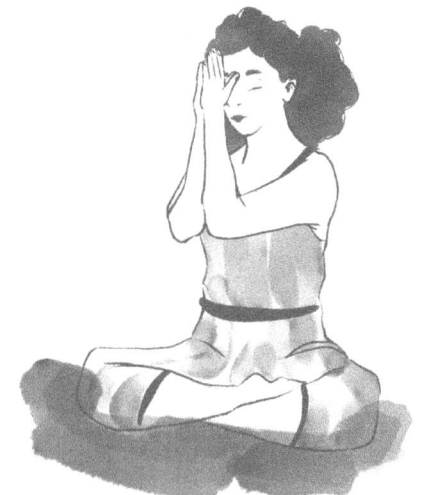

Mudra: Place the hands in Prayer Pose in front of the face. Stretch the thumbs to touch the Third Eye Point.

Eye Focus: Not specified.

Breath: Not specified.

Mantra: Chant the mantra **ARDAAS BHAEE**. (The recording by Anahata Choir was played in the original class.)

**ARDAAS BHAEE, AMAR DAAS GUROO,
AMAR DAAS GUROO, ARDAAS BHAEE,
RAAM DAAS GUROO, RAAM DAAS GUROO,
RAAM DAAS GUROO, SUCHEE SAHEE**

Time: 5 minutes. Immediately begin Part Five.

CONTINUE ON NEXT PAGE »

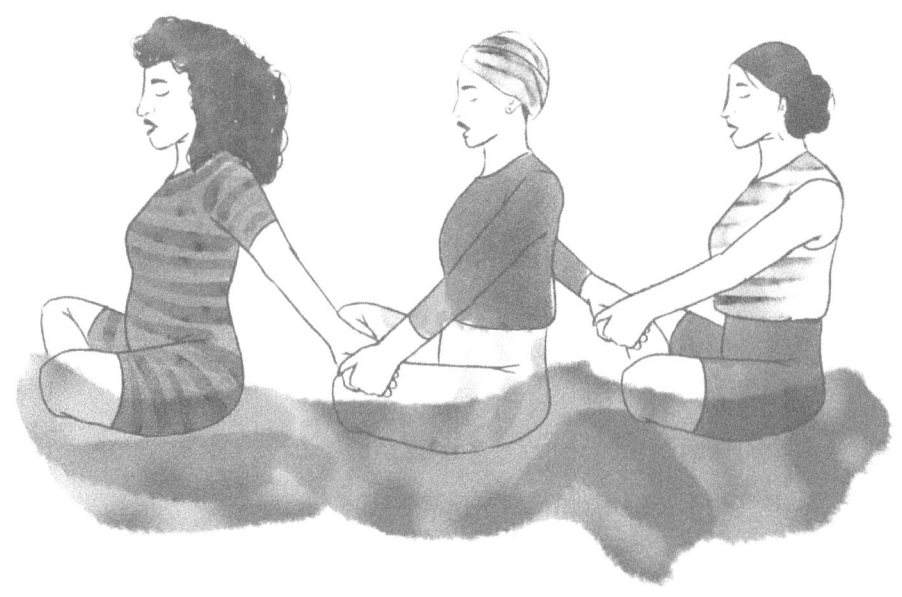

PART FIVE
Remain in Easy Pose.

Mudra & Mantra: Hold hands with the person in front of and behind you, creating a hand chain. (If you are practicing alone, raise one arm forward and the other back, and imagine holding hands to create a chain.) Chant the mantra **ARDAAS BHAEE** for **1 minute**. Meditate on your grace and the flow of loving energy. (The recording by Anahata Choir was played in the original class.) Remain in the posture and silently meditate. Let your touch be healing. Know that the One who created you dwells within you and provides for you. Continue for **1 ½ minutes**.

Eye Focus: Not specified.

Breath: Not specified.

Total Time: 2 ½ minutes.

To End: Inhale deeply and relax.

Comments: If we get into trouble, we can take a deep breath in and hold it for 10, 15, or 20 seconds. With this infusion of praana, we call on our reserve strength; Mother Nature will come through. Call on our reserve force and confront reality.

breathe, rest, concentrate

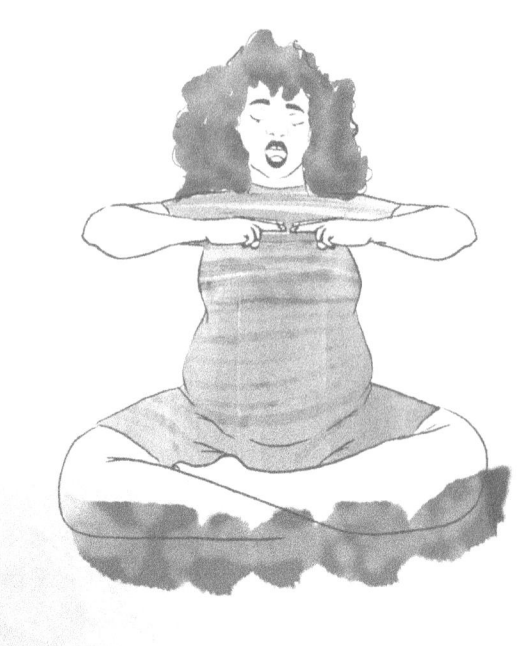

15 / **Kriya to Recognize the God Within**

October 24, 1998

PART ONE
Sit in Easy Pose with a straight spine and a light Neck Lock.

Mudra: Extend the Jupiter (index) and Saturn (middle) fingers on both hands with the other fingers held down with the thumbs. Bring the hands in front of the body at shoulder level, with the elbows out to the sides. The palms are facing down, fingers pointing toward each other with a space between the fingertips.

Eye Focus: Tip of the Nose, looking through the space between the fingers.

Breath: Long Deep Breathing. Inhale through the "O" mouth and exhale through the nose.

Time: 17 minutes.

To End: Inhale deeply, suspend the breath for **15 seconds**, squeeze the spine from the bottom to the top, and Cannon Fire exhale. Inhale deeply, suspend the breath for **20 seconds**, squeeze the spine and the body, and exhale with a whistle. Inhale deeply, suspend the breath for **15 seconds**, squeeze the entire body, and Cannon Fire exhale.

Comments: Relax physically and mentally. It is recommended to urinate after this exercise to eliminate toxins from the body.

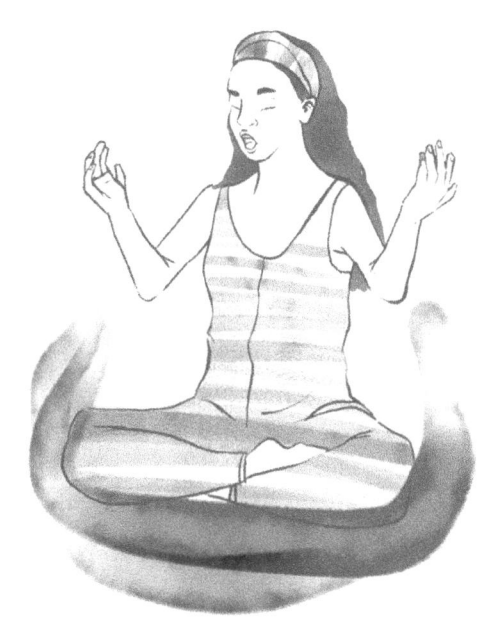

PART TWO
Remain in Easy Pose with a straight spine and a light Neck Lock.

Mudra: Stretch the arms halfway forward with the elbows bent and wider than the shoulders and the forearms angled up slightly. The hands are relaxed.

Eye Focus: Closed.

Breath: Inhale and exhale through the "O" mouth at a pace of one complete breath per 3 seconds. Concentrate on the breath.

Visualization: Imagine you are hugging the Infinite.

Time: 5 minutes.

To End: Inhale deeply, suspend the breath for **10 seconds**, squeeze the body, and Cannon Fire exhale. Repeat **2 more times**. Immediately begin Part Three.

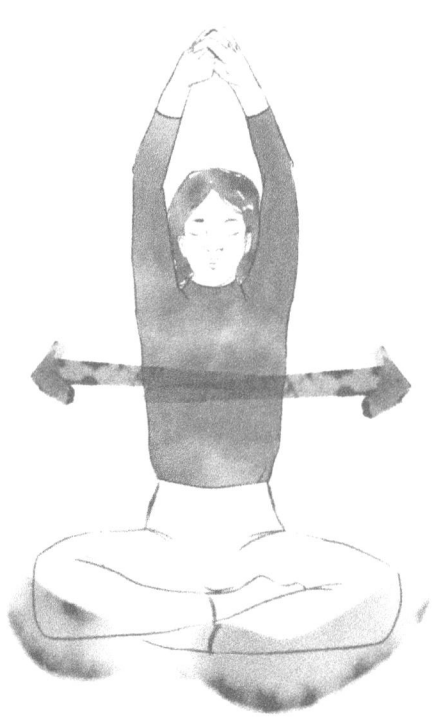

PART THREE

Remain in Easy Pose with a straight spine and a light Neck Lock.

Mudra: Stretch the arms straight up with the hands interlocked. Keeping the arms straight, move the entire spine 3 inches (7-8 cm) to each side. Dance the spine in rhythm with the drums (1 second per cycle).

Eye Focus: Closed.

Breath: Not specified.

Mantra: Chant **HAR** from the navel once per second for the last **3 minutes**.

Time: 11 minutes. (The recording "Pantra" by Mata Mandir Singh was played in the original class.)

To End: Inhale deeply, suspend the breath for **10 seconds**, stretch up powerfully, and exhale. Relax and stretch the arms and body briefly.

PART FOUR

Remain in Easy Pose with a straight spine and a light Neck Lock.

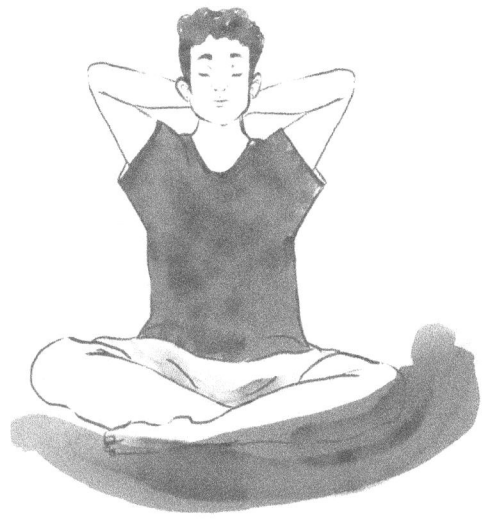

Mudra & Mantra: Interlace the fingers on the back of the neck and stretch the elbows out to the sides. As you chant **HAR** in rhythm with the drums, powerfully draw the elbows in towards each other and back out. Chant **HAR** from the navel twice per second, once as you bring the elbows in and once as you open them out. (The recording "Pantra" by Mata Mandir Singh was played in the original class.)

Eye Focus: Closed.

Breath: Not specified.

Time: 3 minutes.

To End: Inhale deeply, suspend the breath for **10 seconds**, squeeze the body, and exhale. Relax and stretch the body briefly. Immediately begin Part Five.

CONTINUE ON NEXT PAGE »

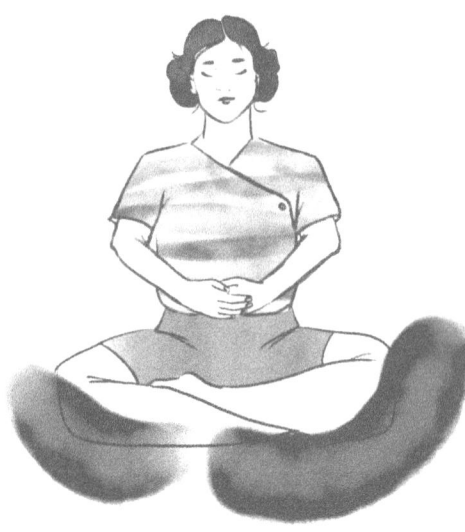

PART FIVE
Remain in Easy Pose.

Mudra: Place the hands on the Navel Point, right on top of the left.

Eye Focus: Closed.

Breath: Long Deep Breathing.

Mantra: Listen and meditate on **RAKHAY RAKHANHAAR**. (The recording by Singh Kaur was played in the original class). Whistle with the music
for the last **6 ½ minutes**.

Time: 13 minutes.

To End: Inhale deeply through the nose, and Cannon
Fire exhale. Repeat **2 more times**.

Comments: Knowledge with experience expands our awareness and elevates our consciousness. We act knowing that God is within us – I am, I am, and all our needs are fulfilled.

*breathe, rest,
concentrate*

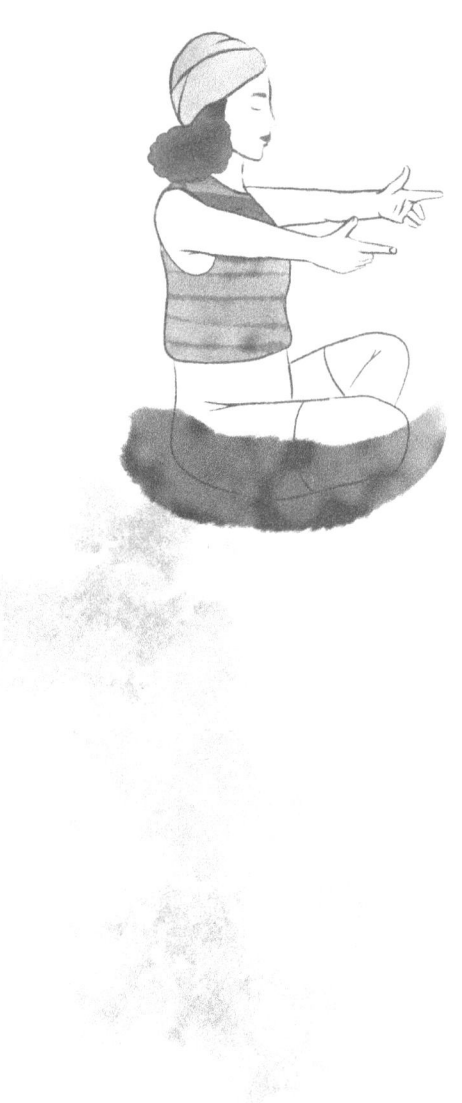

16 / Create a Beam for Opportunity

October 25, 1998

PART ONE
Sit in Easy Pose with a straight spine and a light Neck Lock.

Mudra: Stretch the arms forward parallel to the ground and out at a 60-degree angle from center. Palms face each other with the thumbs pointing up, Jupiter (index) fingers stiff and pointing forward, and the remaining three fingers are bent halfway as if forming a 90-degree angle with the palm.

Eye Focus: Tip of the Nose.

Breath: Inhale deeply through the nose, Cannon Fire exhale through the mouth. Continue for **7 minutes.** Then begin Long Deep Breathing for **2 more minutes**.

Total Time: 9 minutes.

To End: Inhale deeply, suspend the breath for **10 seconds**, and exhale. Immediately begin Part Two.

PART TWO
Remain seated and totally relax the body. Drop the head and shoulders, let the arms be limp.

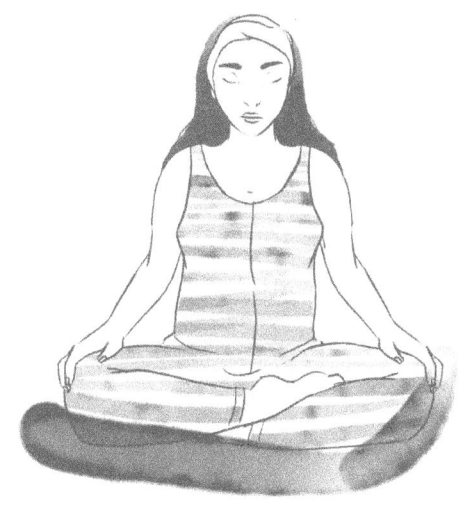

Eye Focus: Not specified.

Breath: Not specified.

Mental Focus: Release and relax; let there be no tension in the body. Let go of control of the body and allow yourself to relax and just be.

Time: 4 minutes.

PART THREE
Remain in Easy Pose with a light Neck Lock.

Mudra: Extend the Jupiter (index) fingers and hold the other fingers down with the thumbs. Bend the elbows closer to the sides of the body and bring the hands to shoulder level with palms facing forward. Curl the Jupiter fingers down on each repetition of **HAR**. Keep the Jupiter fingers up on the other words of the mantra.

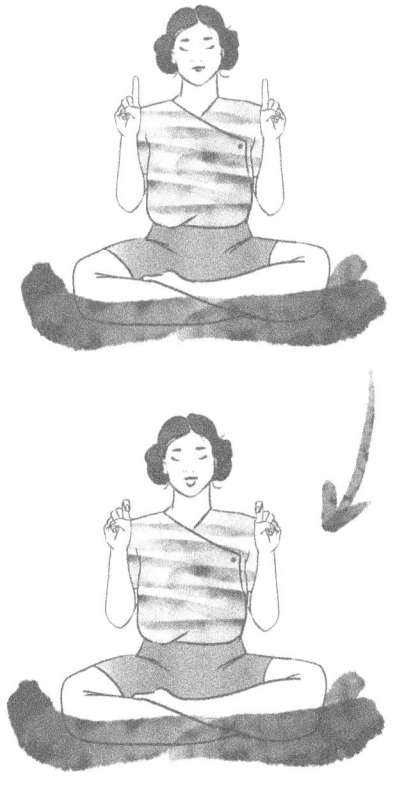

Eye Focus: Not specified.

Breath: Not specified.

CONTINUE ON NEXT PAGE »

Mantra: Chant the Guru Gaitri mantra with **4 HARs**. (The recording "Har Har Har Har Gobinde" by Nirinjan Kaur was played in the original class.)

**HAR HAR HAR HAR GOBINDAY
HAR HAR HAR HAR MUKUNDAY
HAR HAR HAR HAR UDAARAY
HAR HAR HAR HAR APAARAY
HAR HAR HAR HAR HAREEUNG
HAR HAR HAR HAR KAREEUNG
HAR HAR HAR HAR NIRNAAMAY
HAR HAR HAR HAR AKAAMAY**

Time: 12 minutes.

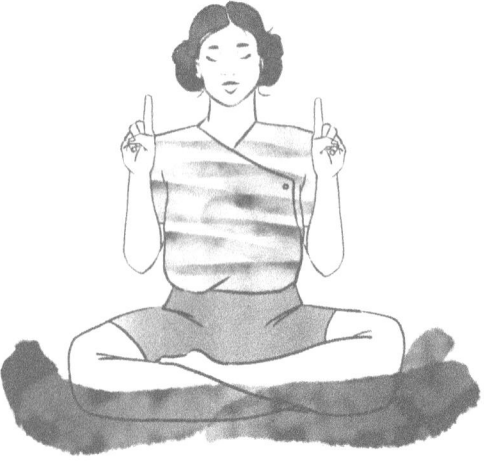

PART FOUR
Remain in Easy Pose.

Mudra: Maintain the mudra from Part Three with Jupiter fingers stiff and straight.

Eye Focus: Not specified.

Breath: Long Deep Breathing through the "O" mouth, filling and emptying the lungs completely with each breath.

Time: 3 minutes.

To End: Inhale deeply, exhale. Totally relax the body as in Part Two.

Comment: It is recommended to urinate after this exercise to release the toxins from the body.

PART FIVE

Sit in Easy Pose with a straight spine and a light Neck Lock.

Mudra: Make an oval with the arms in front of the body at shoulder level, leaving space between the hands. The hands face the body with the thumbs stretched up and the fingers pointing toward each other. Hold the arms, shoulders, neck, and head steady, and maintain the space between the fingers while you dance the spine.

Eye Focus: Closed.

Breath: Not specified.

Mantra: Continue the movement and chant **HAR** from the navel for the last **3 minutes**. (The recording "Pantra" by Mata Mandir Singh was played in the original class.)

Time: 8 ½ minutes.

CONTINUE ON NEXT PAGE »

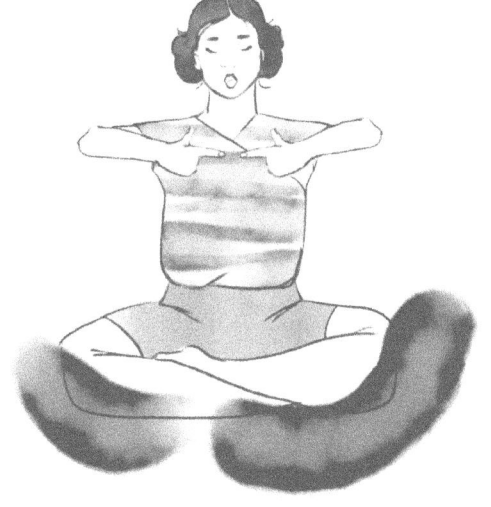

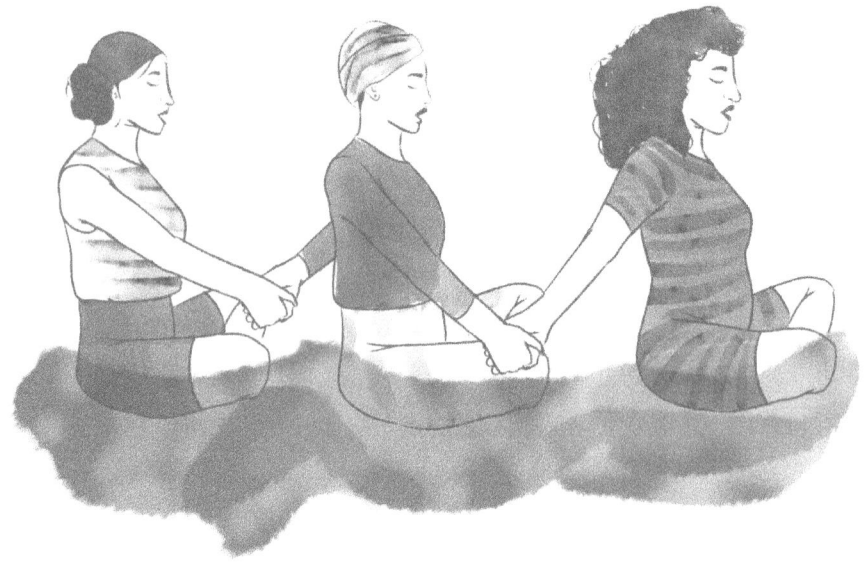

To End: Inhale deeply, hold hands with the people next to you (if practicing alone, imagine that you are holding hands with others), suspend the breath for **15 seconds**, and exhale. Continue holding hands, become thoughtless, and feel the interconnectedness through the flow of the life force. Meditate for **2 minutes**.

Comments: As we expand our awareness through this practice, we can appreciate our own existence. When we appreciate ourselves, we can begin to appreciate the divine, which is not beyond us, but within our existence. With this appreciation, we create a beam that draws opportunity and prosperity toward us.

*breathe, rest,
concentrate*

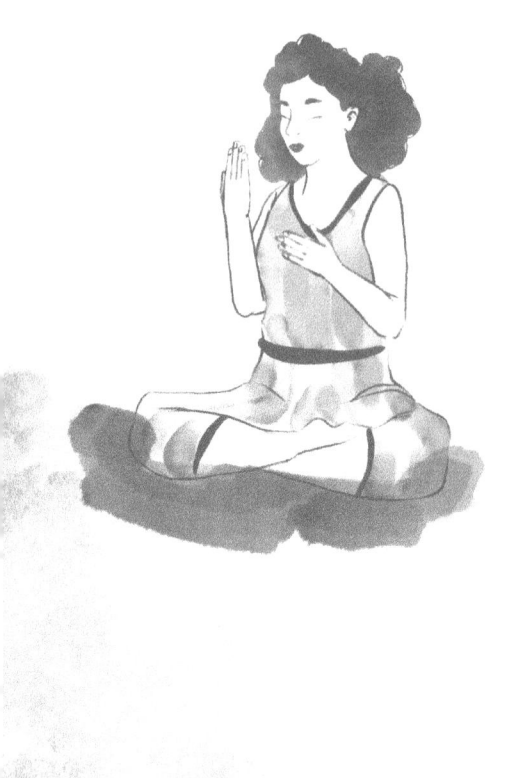

17 / **Come Into Oneness**

November 2, 1998

PART ONE
Sit in Easy Pose with a straight spine and a light Neck Lock.

Mudra: Place the left hand on the Heart Center, with the fingers pointing towards the right. Bring the right hand by the shoulder with the elbow relaxed at the side and the forearm perpendicular to the ground. The palm faces inward, and the fingers point up.

Eye Focus: Closed.

Breath: Long Deep Breathing.

Mental Focus: Rely on the breath of life and go deeply within. Meditate on the Navel Point and find the strength and purity of life in you. Apply self-control and self-knowledge, and have no fear. You are the complete creation of God.

Time: 14 ½ minutes.

To End: Inhale deeply, tighten the fingers, suspend the breath for **20 seconds**, and Cannon Fire exhale Repeat **2 more times**. Relax and talk with others.

PART TWO
Sit in Easy Pose with a straight spine and a light Neck Lock.

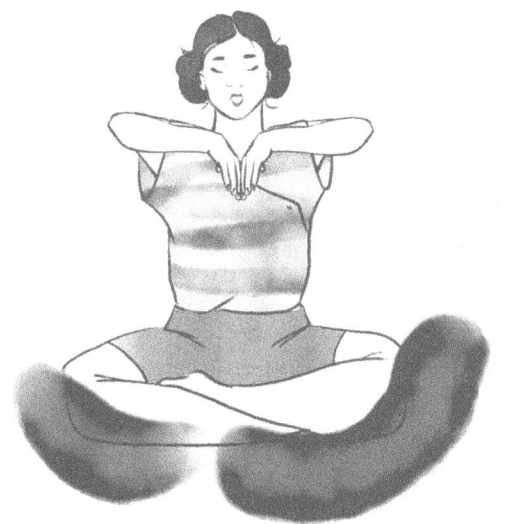

Mudra: Raise the forearms to shoulder level, parallel to the ground, with the elbows bent. Bend the wrists and let the hands hang loose with the backs of the fingers of the opposite hands touching.

Eye Focus: Not specified.

Breath: Long Deep Breathing through the "O" mouth.

Time: 9 ½ minutes.

To End: Continue breathing through the "O" mouth. Inhale deeply, exhale completely, and suspend the breath out for **10 seconds**. Repeat **2 more times**. Immediately begin Part Three.

CONTINUE ON NEXT PAGE »

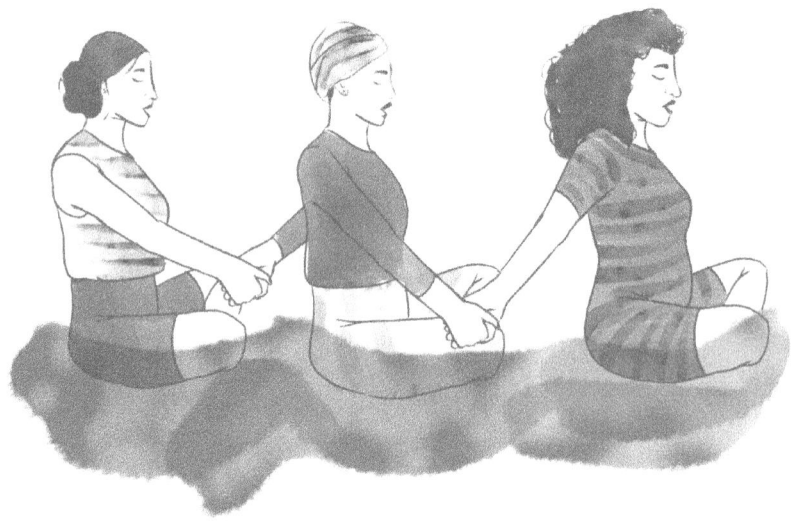

PART THREE
Sit in Easy Pose with a straight spine and a light Neck Lock.

Mudra: Hold hands with the people on either side (if practicing alone, pretend you are holding hands with people.)

Eye Focus: Not specified.

Breath: Cannon Breath.

Time: 2 minutes.

To End: Inhale deeply, suspend the breath for **10 seconds**, squeeze the body, and Cannon Fire exhale. Repeat **2 more times**.

Comments: Long Deep Breathing calls on the reserve energy of the universe. Similarly, holding just one thought of the divine or spirit can bring us out of difficulty in seconds. Give up fascination with things outside ourselves and depending on others. Go deep within and experience oneness with all of creation.

*breathe, rest,
concentrate*

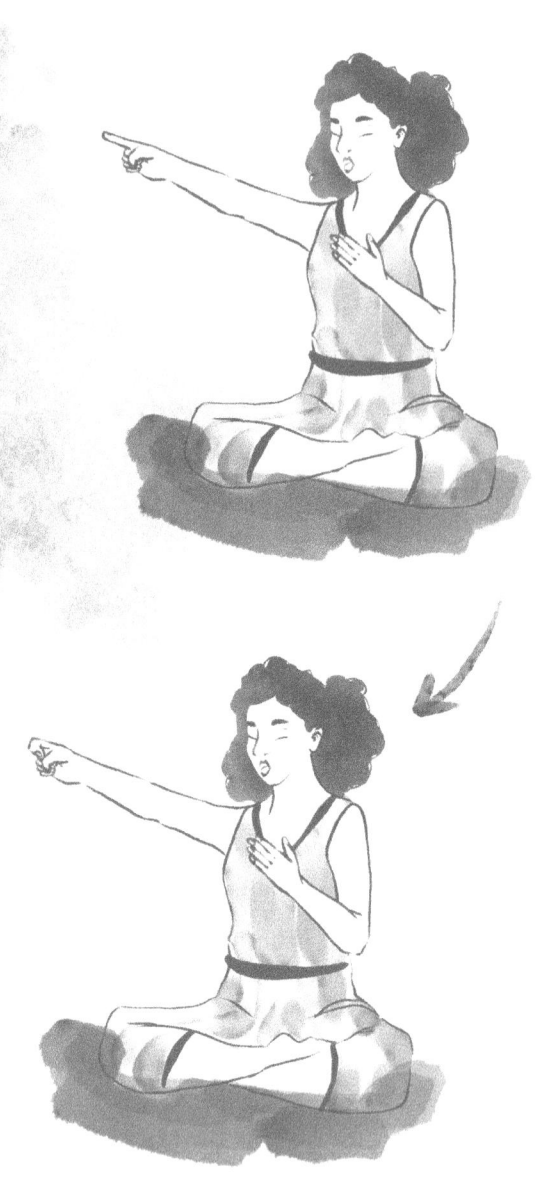

18 / **Reserve Energy to Build Stature**

November 3, 1998

PART ONE
Sit in Easy Pose with a straight spine and a light Neck Lock.

Mudra: Place the left hand on the Heart Center with fingers together, pointing to the right and the thumb relaxed apart. Extend the Jupiter (index) finger of the right hand, with the other fingers held down with the thumb. Stretch the right arm straight forward, 30 degrees above parallel to the ground, with the hand facing down. On the inhale, extend the Jupiter finger, and on the exhale, curl it into the palm.

Eye Focus: Not specified.

Breath: Cannon Breath.

Time: 3 ½ minutes.

To End: Inhale deeply, suspend the breath for **10 seconds**, and powerfully squeeze the Jupiter finger into the palm; exhale and release. Inhale deeply, suspend the breath for **10 seconds**, and very slowly curl the Jupiter finger into the palm; exhale and release. Repeat **1 more time**.

Comments: Breathe strongly to activate the reserve energy.

PART TWO
Remain in Easy Pose with a straight spine and a light Neck Lock.

Mudra: Bring the right hand next to the shoulder with the palm facing forward and the elbow relaxed by the side. Extend the left arm straight forward from the shoulder with the hand facing up, slightly cupped.

Eye Focus: Not specified.

Breath: Inhale through puckered lips in 4, 5, or 6 equal sips as if drinking through a straw, and exhale completely through the nose in one stroke.

Time: 2 minutes.

To End: Inhale deeply, suspend the breath for **15 seconds**, squeeze the entire body, and Cannon Fire exhale. Repeat **2 more** times.

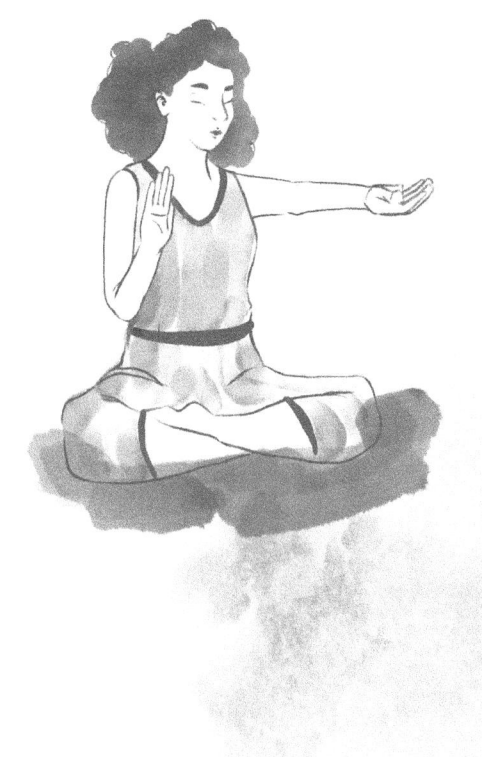

Comments: Stature is a state where our presence is expanded and impactful, we are neutral, and life is harmonious. Without stature, there can be low self-esteem and insecurity. This kriya strengthens the central nervous system, so we have balanced and ample reserve energy. When we can call on our reserve energy to maintain our stature, we can be our authentic selves.

BE YOU

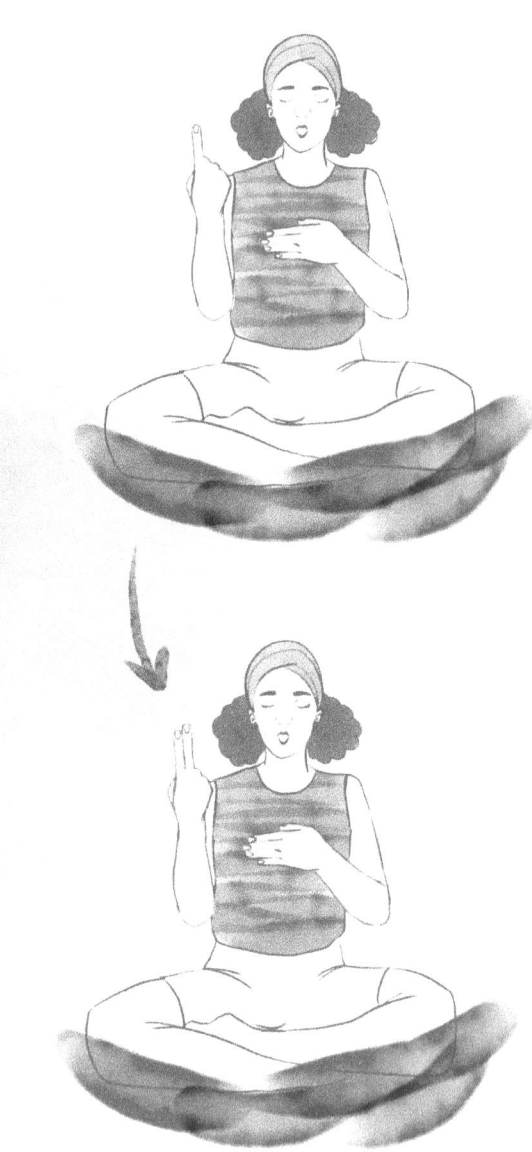

19 / Experience God Within and Find Contentment

November 9, 1998

PART ONE
Sit in Easy Pose with a straight spine and a light Neck Lock.

Mudra: Place the left hand on the Heart Center, with the fingers pointing towards the right. Bring the right hand near the shoulder with the elbow relaxed at the side and the forearm perpendicular to the ground. The palm faces inward, and the fingers point up. Extend the right Jupiter (index) finger and hold the other fingers down with the thumb. On the inhale, release and stretch the Saturn (middle) finger up; on the exhale, curl it down. Keep the Jupiter finger stiff and straight as the other finger moves.

Eye Focus: Not specified.

Breath: Powerfully inhale through the "O" mouth and exhale through the nose.

Time: 10 minutes. Immediately begin Part Two.

PART TWO
Remain in Easy Pose with a straight spine and a light Neck Lock.

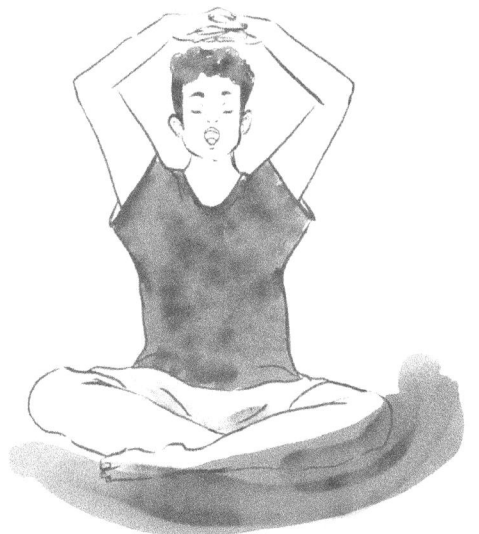

Mudra: Interlace the fingers and raise the arms up, creating an arch above the head with palms facing down.

Eye Focus: Not specified.

Breath: Long Deep Breathing. Inhale through the "O" mouth, exhale through the nose.

Mental Focus: Concentrate on the Heart Center.

Time: 2 ½ minutes. Immediately begin Part Three.

CONTINUE ON NEXT PAGE »

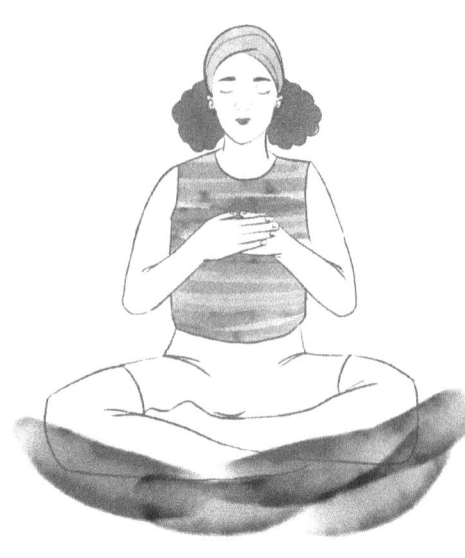

PART THREE
Remain in Easy Pose with a straight spine and a light Neck Lock.

Mudra: Place the hands on the Heart Center, right over left.

Eye Focus: Not specified.

Breath: Long Deep Breathing.

Mental Focus: Find God with your heart. Imagine God sitting in your Heart Center, and be aware of the breath of life as a most precious prayer.

Time: 10 minutes.

To End: Hold and lock the elbows with the opposite hands. Inhale deeply, suspend the breath for **20 seconds**, squeeze the body, and Cannon fire exhale. Repeat **2 more times**.

Comments: In the Aquarian Age, we recognize that God is not in heaven but within us. The more open and authentic we are, the more God emanates from our hearts. The experience of this reality brings contentment to our lives.

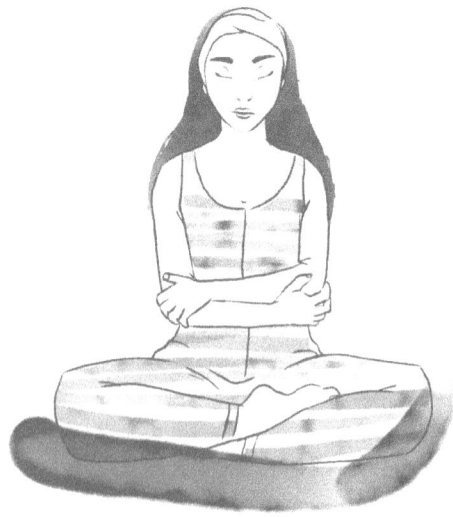

breathe, rest, concentrate

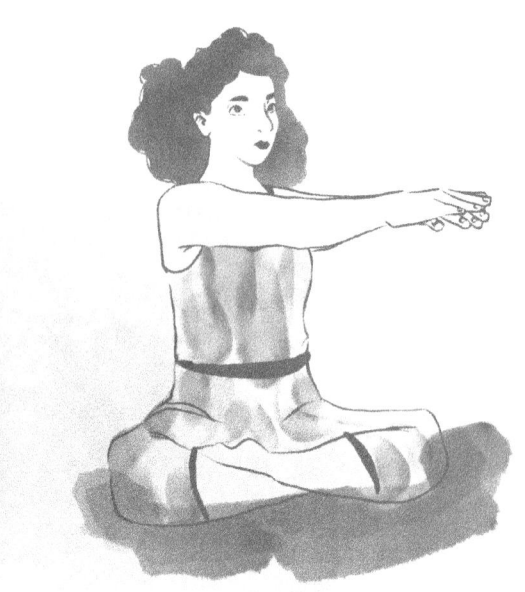

20 / Open the Heart to Experience Yourself

December 17, 1998

PART ONE
Sit in Easy Pose with a straight spine and a light Neck Lock.

Mudra: Stretch the arms forward from the shoulders and raise the forearms 1 inch (3 cm) above shoulder level, keeping them parallel to the ground. Place the right hand on top of the left, palms facing down, and the heel of the right hand on top of the heel of the left hand.

Eye Focus: Stare straight ahead over the arms.

Breath: Long Deep Breathing. Inhale through the "O" mouth and exhale through the nose.

Time: 10 minutes.

To End: Inhale deeply, suspend the breath for **15 seconds**, squeeze the entire body, and Cannon Fire exhale. Repeat **2 more times**; the last time, slowly exhale.

PART TWO
Remain in Easy Pose with a straight spine and a light Neck Lock.

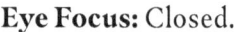

Mudra: Place the pad of the right Jupiter (index) finger on the pad of the left index finger, creating a 45-degree angle, with the right palm facing down and the left palm facing up. The other fingers are curled into the palms with thumbs holding them down. Hold the mudra relaxed in front of the body with the forearms parallel to the ground.

Eye Focus: Closed.

Breath: Not specified.

Mantra: HAR. Listen and pump the navel powerfully on each repetition of the mantra. (The recording "Tantric Har" by Simran Kaur and Guru Prem Singh was played in the original class.)

Time: 15 minutes. Immediately begin Part Three.

Comments: Pumping the navel powerfully moves the shoulders, ribcage and spine.

CONTINUE ON NEXT PAGE »

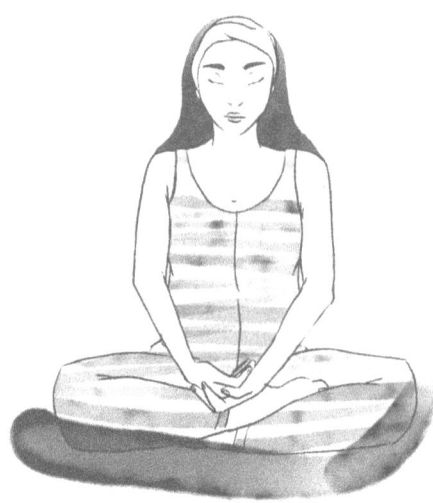

PART THREE
Remain in Easy Pose.

Mudra: Relax the hands in the lap.

Eye Focus: Not specified.

Breath: Cannon Breath.

Time: 1 minute.

To End: Inhale deeply, suspend the breath for **15 seconds**, squeeze the body, starting from the base of the spine to the top of the head, and exhale. Repeat **2 more times**.

Comments: Open the heart in this kriya to experience ourselves, to know from experience that God is within us. When we act and speak out of that knowing, we are naturally compassionate, careful, and true to our values. We are not the body, mind, or spirit, but the one who holds those parts together.

21 / Open the Heart Center and See Life as a Gift

December 20, 1998

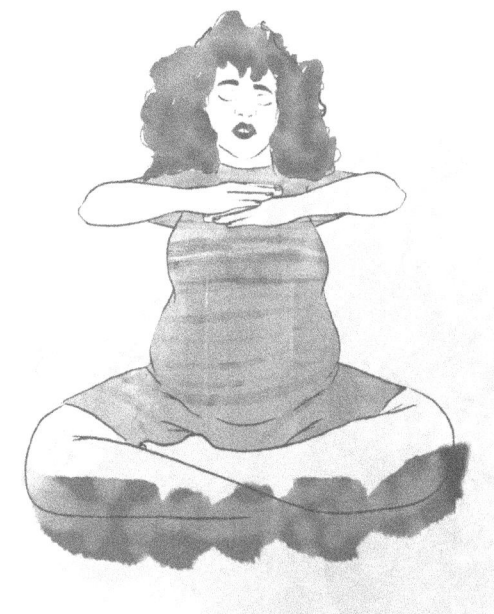

PART ONE
Sit in Easy Pose with a straight spine and a light Neck Lock.

Mudra: Bring the hands in front of the body at shoulder level, with the elbows out to the sides. Place the right hand on top of the left, both palms facing down, and cross the thumbs to lock them, keeping the arms parallel to the ground.

Eye Focus: Not specified.

Breath: Inhale through the mouth and exhale through the nose for the first **1 minute.**

Mantra: Chant **HAR**, pulling in the Navel Point with each repetition. (The "Tantric Har" recording by Simran Kaur and Guru Prem Singh was played in the original class.)

Time: 11 minutes.

To End: Inhale deeply, suspend the breath for **15 seconds**, squeeze the entire body, distribute the energy, and Cannon Fire exhale.

Repeat **1 more time**. Inhale deeply, suspend the breath for **30 seconds**, squeeze the spine from the base to the top, and Cannon Fire exhale.

CONTINUE ON NEXT PAGE »

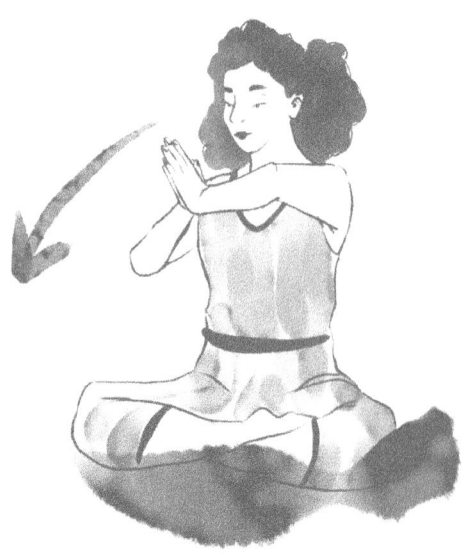

PART TWO
Remain in Easy Pose with a straight spine and a light Neck Lock.

Mudra: Place the palms together in Prayer Pose in front of the right shoulder, fingers pointing up. The left elbow is raised so that the forearm is parallel to the ground, and the right elbow is relaxed down. Rotate the hands forward and back from the wrists each time you chant **HAR**.

Eye Focus: Not specified.

Breath: Not specified.

Mantra: Chant **HAR** from the navel. (The recording "Tantric Har" by Simran Kaur and Guru Prem Singh was played in the original class.)

Time: 5 minutes.

To End: Inhale deeply, squeeze the body, press the palms together, suspend the breath for **20 seconds**, and exhale. Repeat **2 more times**; the last time, exhale with a whistle. Immediately begin Part Three.

PART THREE
Remain in Easy Pose.

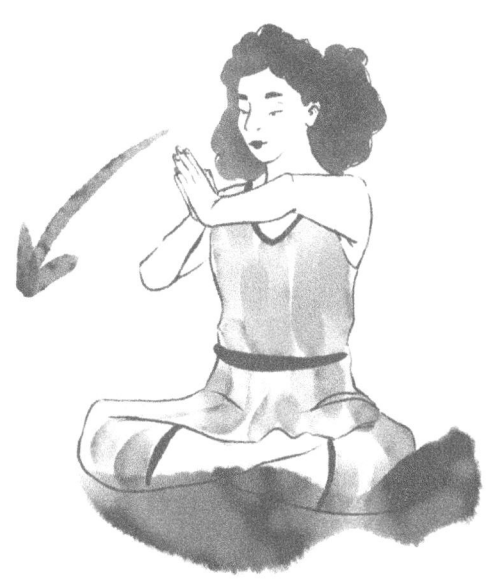

Mudra: Maintain the same mudra as in Part Two.

Eye Focus: Not specified.

Breath: Not specified.

Mantra: Whistle **ARDAS BHAEE**. (The instrumental version from the album *Healing Sounds of the Ancients* #5 was played in the original class.)

Time: 4 minutes.

To End: Inhale deeply, exhale, then sit in silence for **1 minute** with Long Deep Breathing. Pray to your soul, befriend your soul, and promise that you will not neglect your soul.

Comments: An open heart sees that life is a gift and that the breath, Pavan Guru, sustains us. Through our personality, our identity, we hold the body, mind, and soul until death, when the body and mind dissolve and the soul departs on its journey.

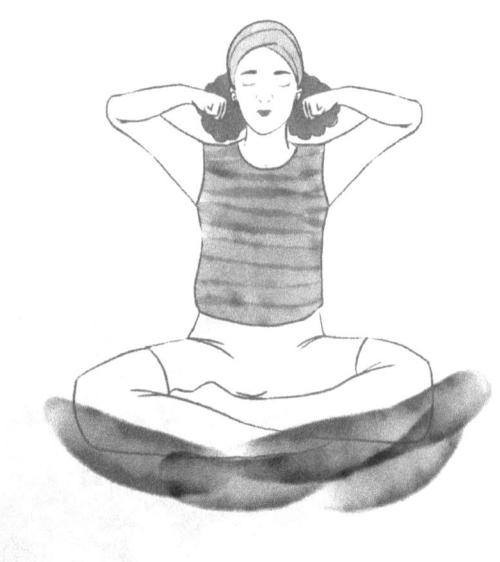

22 / **For Clarity of Mind**

December 28, 1998

PART ONE
Sit in Easy Pose with a straight spine and light Neck Lock.

Mudra: Make fists, bringing them above the shoulders with the elbows out to the sides and the palms facing down. Keep the arms up and the fists tight.

Eye Focus: Tip of the Nose.

Breath: Long Deep Breathing. Sip the air in through puckered lips and exhale through the nose.

Time: 11 minutes.

To End: Inhale deeply, suspend the breath for **10 seconds**, tighten the body, and Cannon Fire exhale. Repeat **2 more times**.

Comments: This exercise works on the frontal lobe of the brain.

PART TWO
Sit in Easy Pose with a straight spine and a light Neck Lock.

Mudra & Breath: With the elbows out to the sides, bring the hands relaxed in front of the chest, with the palms facing down and fingers separated. As you inhale through the nose with great tension, close the fingers into tight fists, drop the arms, and roll the shoulders back and up toward the ears. As you Cannon Fire exhale, quickly release the arms and return to the starting position.

Eye Focus: Not specified.

Time: 5 minutes.

To End: Inhale deeply, raise the shoulders as high as possible, tighten the fists and arms, suspend the breath for **10 seconds**, and exhale. Repeat **2 more times**.

Comments: This exercise breaks up the deposits in the shoulders and adjusts the spine.

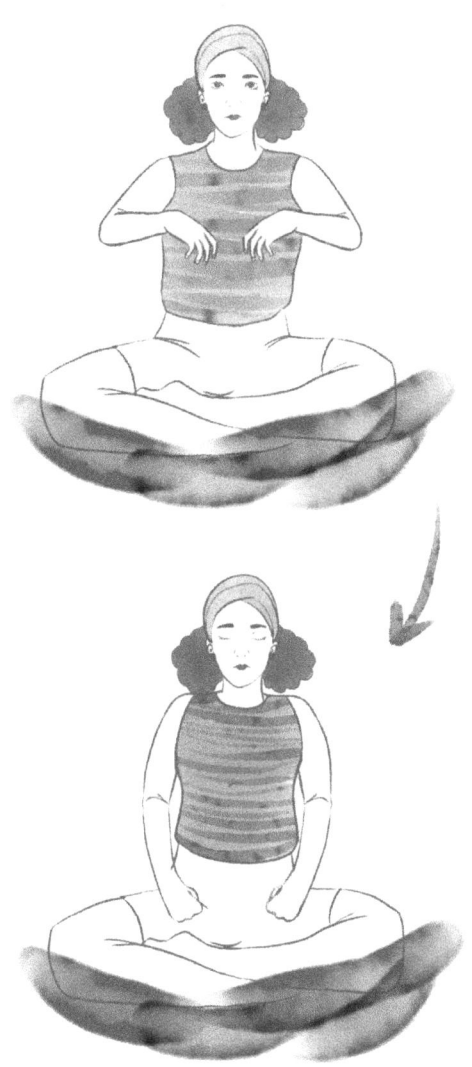

BE YOU

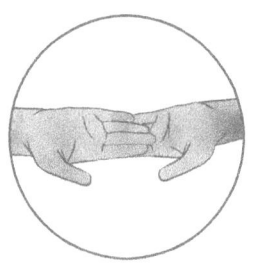
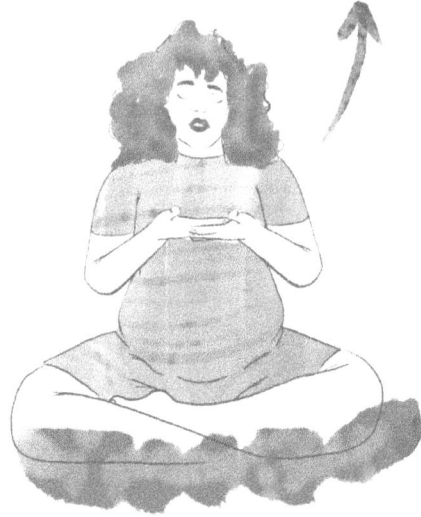

PART THREE

Sit in Easy Pose with a straight spine and a light Neck Lock.

Mudra: Place the hands in front of the chest with the palms facing up, right hand fingers crossed on top of the left hand fingers, thumbs stretched away from the hand, and elbows relaxed by the sides of the body.

Eye Focus: Closed.

Breath: Not specified.

Mantra: Pull the navel strongly as you chant **HAR** once per second; the shoulders will move with the movement of the navel. (The recording "Tantric Har" by Simran Kaur and Guru Prem Singh was played in the original class.)

Time: 4 minutes.

To End: Inhale deeply, suspend the breath for **10 seconds**, pull the navel in strongly, and Cannon Fire exhale. Repeat **2 more times**.

Comments: Clarity is the beauty of the mind. As we practice this kriya, unconscious thoughts may first come up and then vanish, clearing the mind.

breathe, rest, concentrate

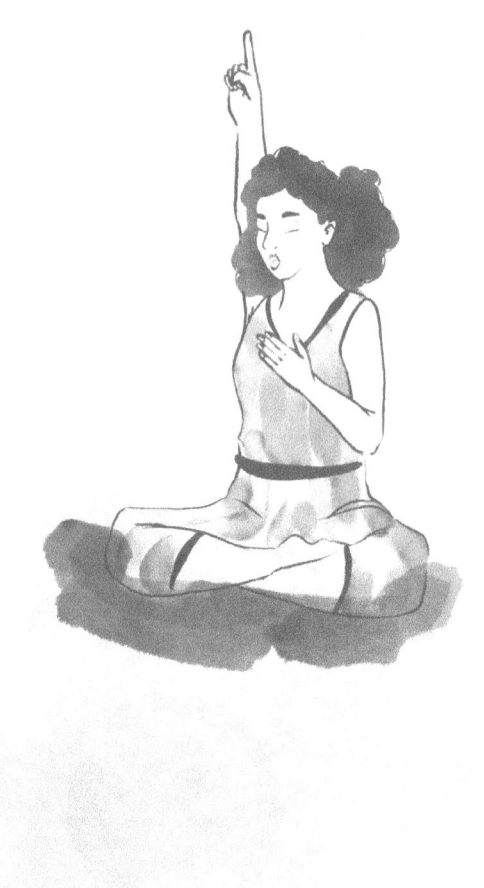

23 / **Meditation for Subtlety and Intuition**

January 18, 1999

Sit in Easy Pose with a straight spine and a light Neck Lock.

Mudra: Place the left palm on the Heart Center. Extend the right Jupiter (index) finger and hold the other fingers down with the thumb. Stretch the right arm straight up, close to the ear, palm facing forward.

Eye Focus: Not specified

Breath: Long Deep Breathing. Inhale through the "O" mouth and exhale through the nose.

Mantra: Listen to the mantra **RAKHAY RAKHANHAAR**. (The recording by Singh Kaur was played in the original class.)

RAKHAY RAKHANHAAR AAP UBAARIUN
GUR KEE PAIREE PAA-EH KAAJ SAVAARIUN
HOAA AAP DAYAAL MANHO NA VISAARIUN
SAADH JANAA KAI SUNG BHAVJAL TAARIUN
SAAKAT NINDAK DUSHT KHIN MAA-EH BIDAARIUN
TIS SAAHIB KEE TAYK NAANAK MANAI MAA-EH
JIS SIMRAT SUKH HO-EH SAGLAY DOOKH JAA-EH

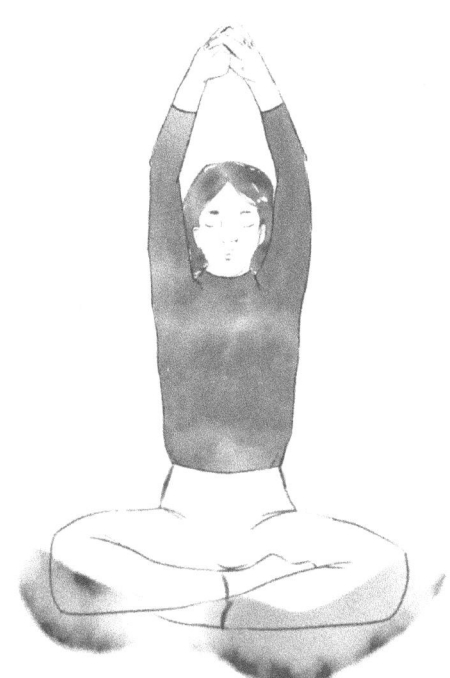

Time: 18 minutes.

To End: Interlock the fingers and stretch the arms up above the head. Inhale deeply, suspend the breath for **15 seconds**, and Cannon Fire exhale. Repeat **2 more times**.

Comments: At death, the soul is carried by the subtle body on its journey beyond. It is possible and desirable to experience the subtle body while alive, rather than being attached only to the physical body and the mind. When the subtle body penetrates through the material world, through intuition, we know who we really are.

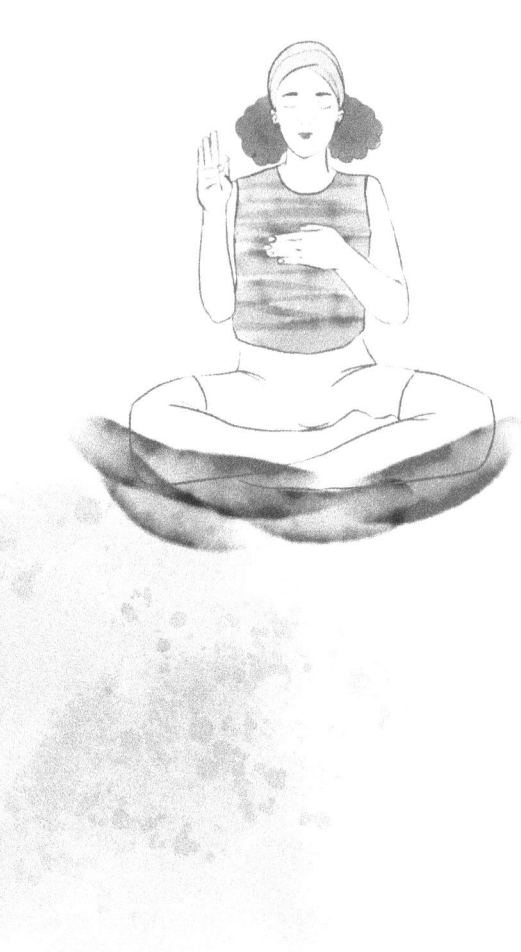

24 / Control Your Thoughts

January 20, 1999

Sit in Easy Pose with a straight spine and a light Neck Lock.

Mudra: Place the left hand on the Heart Center. Bring the right hand by the shoulder, touching the tip of the thumb to the tip of the Jupiter (index) finger in Gyan Mudra with the palm facing forward. Control your mind and become thoughtless.

Eye Focus: Closed.

Breath: Not specified.

Time: 11 minutes.

To End: Inhale deeply, suspend the breath for **15 seconds**, and exhale. Repeat **2 more times**, squeezing all the muscles of the body tightly on the last hold.

Comments: All human action begins as thoughts. When we attach ourselves to a thought and it becomes a wish or a fantasy, that thought gets stretched out. In this kriya, we practice thoughtlessness, so that we no longer expand our thoughts. When we develop the habit of not stretching our thoughts, we receive clear guidance and act from our intuition.

breathe, rest, concentrate

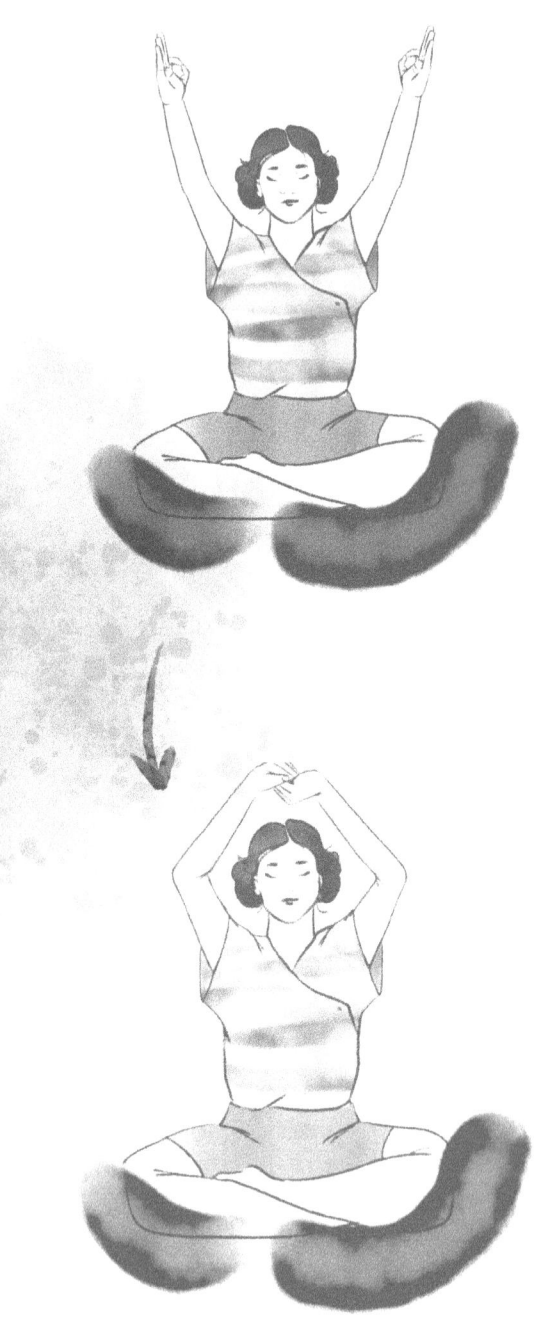

25 / **Energize the Brain**

January 26, 1999

Sit in Easy Pose with a straight spine and a light Neck Lock.

Mudra: Touch the tips of the thumbs and the Jupiter (index) fingers in Gyan Mudra, and keep the other fingers straight. Bring the arms up and out to the sides at a 60-degree angle with palms facing up. Stretch out from the shoulders and elbows strongly.

Eye Focus: Not specified.

Breath: Inhale in 4 strokes through the "O" mouth and exhale in 4 strokes through the "O" mouth.

Time: 11 minutes.

To End: Hook the fingers together above the head in Bear Grip, with the right palm facing down and the left facing up. Inhale deeply, suspend the breath for **10 seconds**, pull strongly on the grip, and Cannon Fire exhale. Repeat **1 time**.

Comments: Human life is a gift. With regular meditation practice, we develop a clear mind; we see, understand, believe, trust, and act consciously. We can find ourselves and merge with our higher Self.

*breathe, rest,
concentrate*

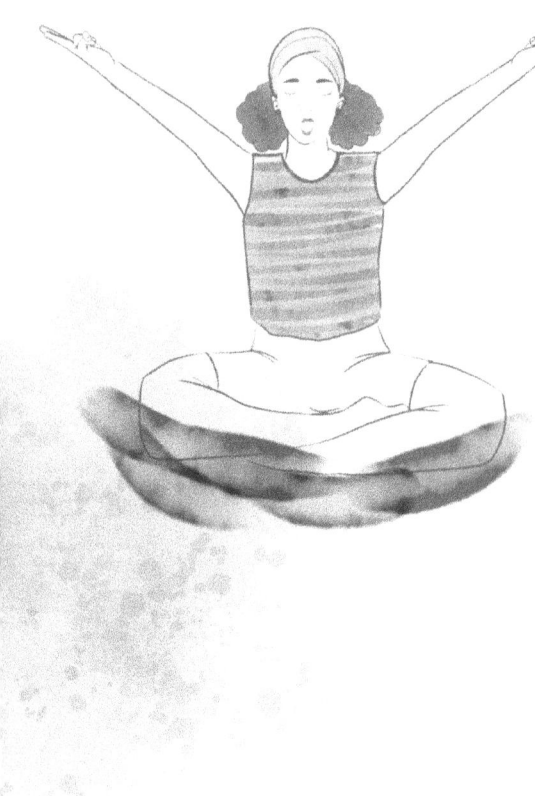

26 / **Change Your Electromagnetic Field**

January 27, 1999

Sit in Easy Pose with a straight spine and a light Neck Lock.

Mudra: Extend the Jupiter (index) and Saturn (middle) fingers and hold the other fingers down with the thumb. Bring the arms up and out to the sides at a 60-degree angle with palms facing up. Stretch out from the shoulders and elbows strongly.

Eye Focus: Not specified.

Breath: Through the "O" mouth. Inhale in 4 strokes and exhale in 4 strokes.

Time: 11 minutes.

To End: Stretch the arms above the head with palms facing forward, fingers together and thumbs relaxed. Alternatively move the arms up and down very fast for **1 minute**. Inhale deeply and interlace the fingers above the head, stretch up, suspend the breath for **10 seconds**, and exhale. Repeat **1 time**.

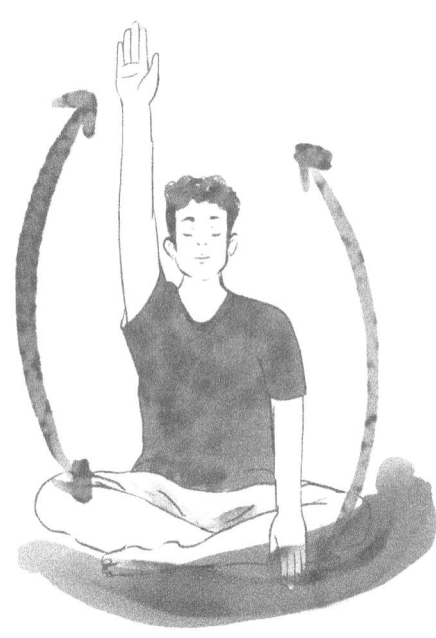

Comments: This kriya can build our electromagnetic field and expand our being. Emotions like fear limit us, causing us to react, which results in consequences, or karma. With our sensory system, we experience infinity in the present moment and avoid karma by acting naturally and clearly.

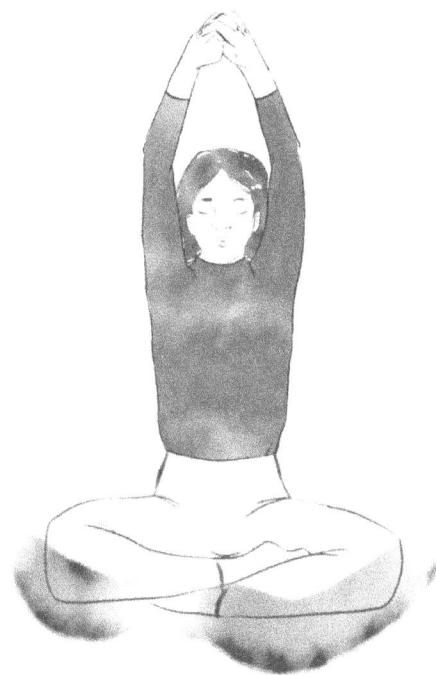

27 / Resolve Inner Anger To Be Happy

February 2, 1999

Sit in Easy Pose with a straight spine and a light Neck Lock.

Mudra: Stretch the arms out to the sides parallel to the ground with fingers together and palms facing down. Keeping the arms straight, move the hands up and down from the wrists twice per word of the mantra.

Eye Focus: Closed.

Breath: Not specified.

Mantra: Listen to the Guru Gaitri mantra with **4 HARs**. (The recording by Nirinjan Kaur from *White Tantra Volume 1* was played in the original class.)

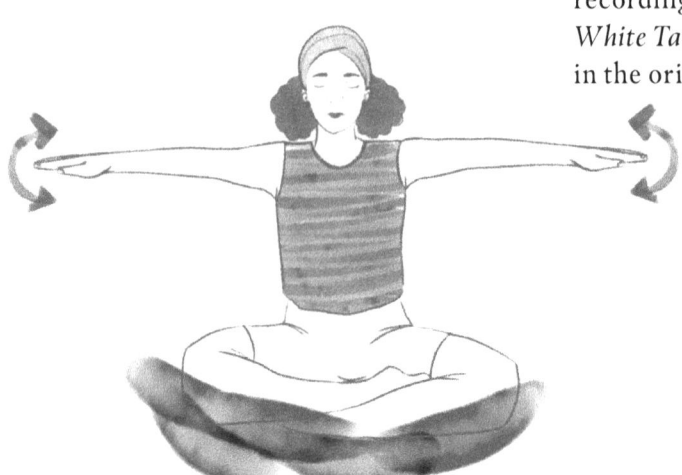

**HAR HAR HAR HAR
GOBINDAY
HAR HAR HAR HAR
MUKUNDAY
HAR HAR HAR HAR
UDAARAY
HAR HAR HAR HAR
APAARAY
HAR HAR HAR HAR
HAREEUNG
HAR HAR HAR HAR
KAREEUNG
HAR HAR HAR HAR
NIRNAAMAY
HAR HAR HAR HAR
AKAAMAY**

Time: 11 minutes.

To End: Inhale deeply, suspend the breath for **10 seconds**, move the hands from the wrists very fast and squeeze the body, and then exhale. Repeat **2 more times**.

Comments: We all experience disappointments throughout life, from birth to adulthood. If we don't deal with the resulting emotion, this sadness turns into frozen inner anger. When we don't acknowledge our inner anger, we feel that we cannot achieve, and then we become insecure. This insecurity can cause outbursts, a lack of trust in others, and isolation. The way to be happy is to stop the fantasy, the lies we tell ourselves based on our insecurity, and recognize our reality.

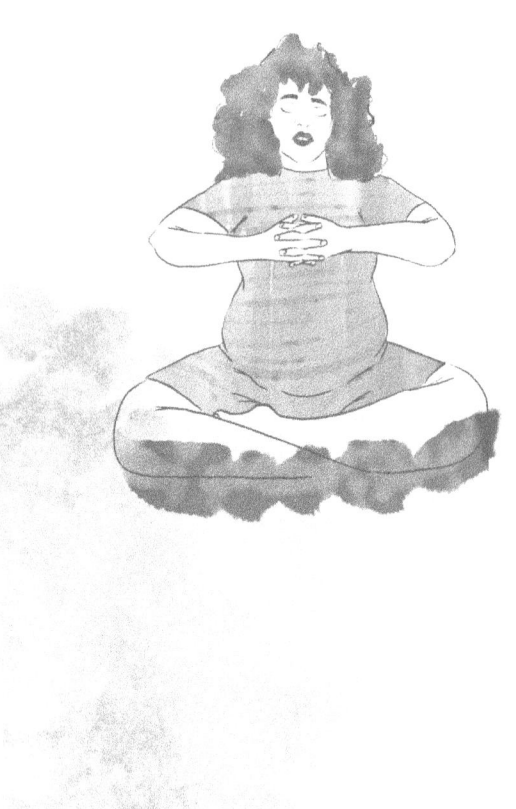

28 / Flow of Prosperity

February 9, 1999

Sit in Easy Pose with a straight spine and a light Neck Lock.

Mudra: Interlock the hands at the level of the Heart Center with palms facing the body and forearms parallel to the ground. Pull the hands strongly without separating them.

Eye Focus: Closed.

Breath: Not specified.

Mantra: Chant the Guru Gaitri mantra with **4 HARs**. (The recording "Har Har Har Har Gobinde" by Nirinjan Kaur from *White Tantra Volume 1* was played in the original class.)

HAR HAR HAR HAR
GOBINDAY
HAR HAR HAR HAR
MUKUNDAY
HAR HAR HAR HAR
UDAARAY
HAR HAR HAR HAR
APAARAY
HAR HAR HAR HAR
HAREEUNG
HAR HAR HAR HAR
KAREEUNG
HAR HAR HAR HAR
NIRNAAMAY
HAR HAR HAR HAR
AKAAMAY

Time: 11 minutes.

To End: Inhale deeply, suspend the breath for **15 seconds**, pull the hands forcefully, and exhale. Repeat **2 more times.** On the last suspension, bring the mudra to the level of the eyes.

Comments: Without trust in God, we can become angry, jealous, and insecure. We try to discharge our anger and emotions through distractions, denying ourselves. All that is needed is to be ourselves and find God's presence within us. We can rest comfortably and gratefully in this flow of prosperity, which is grace.

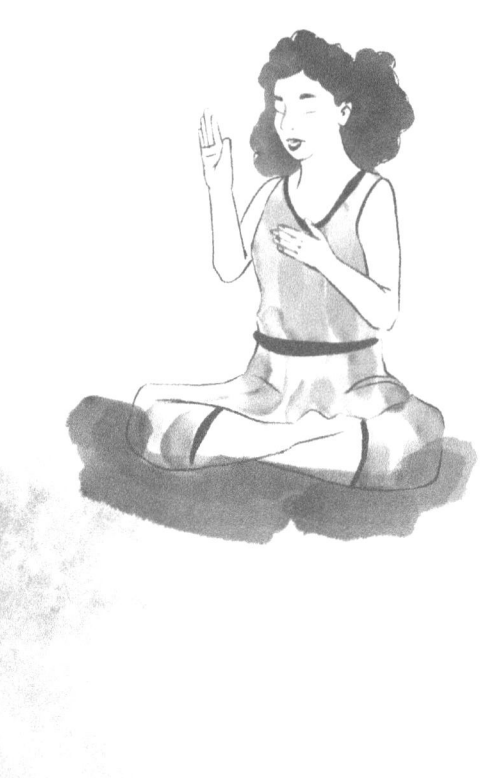

29 / **Bless All Beings**

February 15, 1999

PART ONE
Sit in Easy Pose with a straight spine and a light Neck Lock.

Mudra: Place the left palm on the Heart Center. Raise the right hand above shoulder level, palm facing forward, with the arm extended slightly forward. Bless the earth and all beings.

Eye Focus: Closed.

Breath: Not specified.

Mantra: Chant **WHAA-HAY GUROO WHAA-HAY JEEO**. (The recording by Harjinder Singh Gill and Sangeet Kaur Khalsa from the album *Raga Sadhana* was played in the original class.)

Time: 15 minutes.

To End: Inhale, exhale, and immediately begin Part Two.

PART TWO
Remain in the posture.

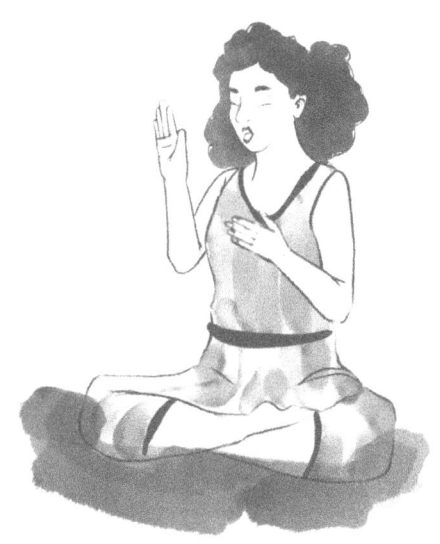

Mudra: Maintain the same mudra as in Part One.

Eye Focus: Closed.

Breath: Inhale and exhale through the "O" mouth as fast as you can. Breathe with the diaphragm.

Time: 1 ½ minutes.

To End: Inhale deeply, stretch the arms up with hands open and fingers open wide and stiff. Shake only the hands from the wrist, suspend the breath for **15 seconds**, and exhale. Repeat **2 more times**.

Comments: During challenges in life, we can rise above the commotion by fixing our attention on the Infinite to ride out the storm.

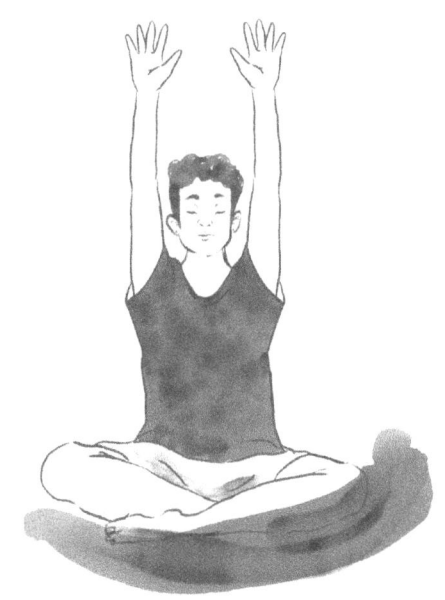

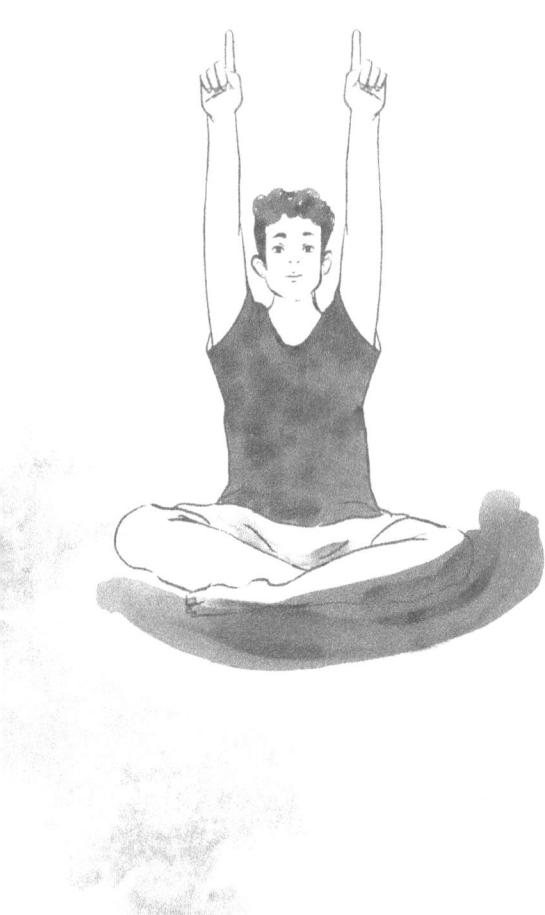

30 / **Forgive to Be Authentic and Honest**

February 16, 1999

Sit in Easy Pose with a straight spine and a light Neck Lock.

Mudra: Extend the Jupiter (index) fingers and curl the other fingers down. Stretch the arms straight up with palms facing forward and the Jupiter finger pointing up.

Eye Focus: Closed.

Breath: Not specified.

Mantra: Chant **WHAA-HAY GUROO WHAA-HAY JEEO** from the navel. (The recording by Sangeet Kaur from the album *Raga Sadhana* was played in the original class.)

Time: 18 minutes.

To End: Keeping the arms raised overhead, interlock the Jupiter (index) fingers, inhale deeply, pull on the fingers strongly, squeeze the entire body, suspend the breath for **15 seconds**, and exhale. Interlock the Saturn (middle) fingers, inhale deeply, suspend the breath for **10 seconds**, pull on the fingers strongly, squeeze the entire body, and exhale. Interlock the Sun (ring) fingers, inhale deeply, suspend the breath for **15 seconds**, pull on the fingers strongly, squeeze the entire body, and exhale.

Comments: When we don't have proper support and guidance in life, inner anger builds, and we lack the security to mature. Anger motivates us, and we feel deficient and are afraid our weaknesses will be seen. The solution is forgiveness—forgiving ourselves, then we are able to forgive others. We can then be authentically honest in all relationships.

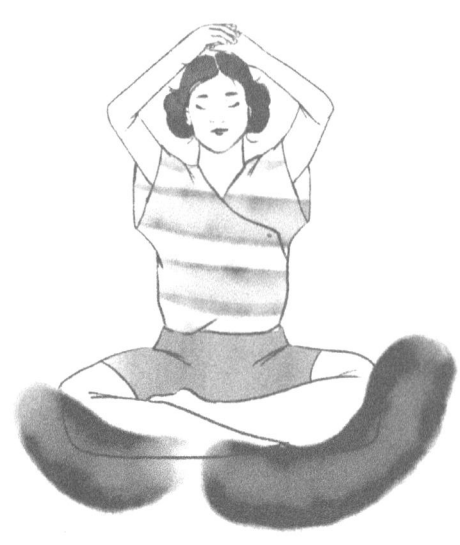

31 / Meditation for Manifestation

DHARAM VISRAN KRIYA
February 22, 1999

Sit in Easy Pose with a straight spine and a light Neck Lock.

Mudra: Place the right hand on top of the left with palms facing down, slightly cupped. Create an arc with the arms, holding the hands in front of the top of the head.

Eye Focus: Closed.

Mantra:
a) Chant the mantra **Guru Ram Das Teri Saran** for **14 minutes**,
b) Do Breath of Fire for **5 minutes**,
c) Chant the mantra again for **12 minutes**. (The recording by Bhai Sadhu Singh Dehradun was played during the original class.)

Total Time: 31 minutes.

To End: Inhale deeply, hold the posture, suspend the breath for **10 seconds**, squeeze the body, direct all the pressure to the hands, and exhale. Repeat **2 more times**.

Comments: In this kriya, the sound and the Self merge. What we hear and say is the will of God. Our will and God's will are one.

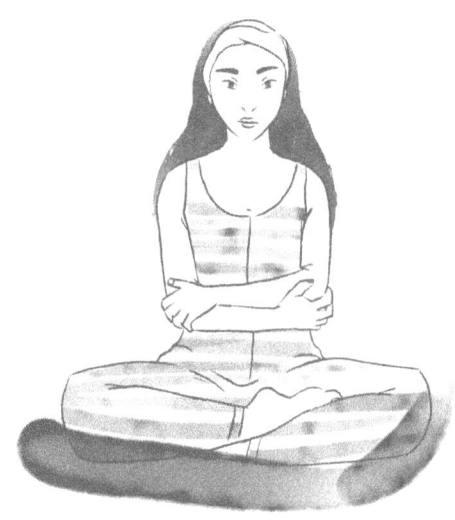

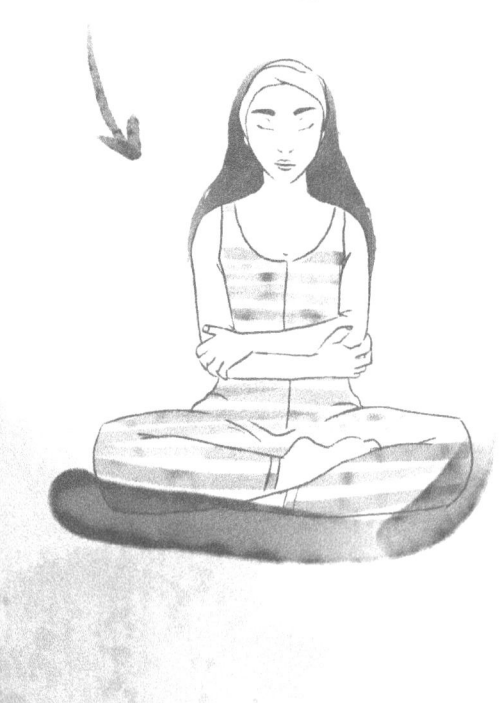

32 / **Be Your True Self**

February 23, 1999

Sit in Easy Pose with a straight spine and a light Neck Lock.

Mudra: Grasp the opposite elbow with each hand and rest the arms on the body.

Eye Focus: Open in part a) and closed in part b).

Mantra and Breath:
a) Chant **RAKHAY RAKHANHAAR** from the navel for **13 minutes**. (The recording by Singh Kaur was played in the original class.)

**RAKHAY RAKHANHAAR AAP UBAARIUN
GUR KEE PAIREE PAA-EH KAAJ SAVAARIUN
HOAA AAP DAYAAL MANHO NA VISAARIUN
SAADH JANAA KAI SUNG BHAVJAL TAARIUN
SAAKAT NINDAK DUSHT KHIN MAA-EH BIDAARIUN
TIS SAAHIB KEE TAYK NAANAK MANAI MAA-EH
JIS SIMRAT SUKH HO-EH SAGLAY DOOKH JAA-EH**

b) Long Deep Breathing. Listen to the shabad **GURU SATGURU KA JO SIKH AKHAYE**, and sense its effects for **5 minutes**. (The recording "Hukam" by Singh Kaur was played in the original class.)

Total Time: 18 minutes.

Comments: Inner anger builds up underneath our protective shell or persona. It bursts out unexpectedly, hurting others and ourselves. Instead of getting angry and projecting it onto others, we can face ourselves. The more we express our true selves, the power and beauty of our soul shine through, and we live in our innocence. Then Mother Nature serves us.

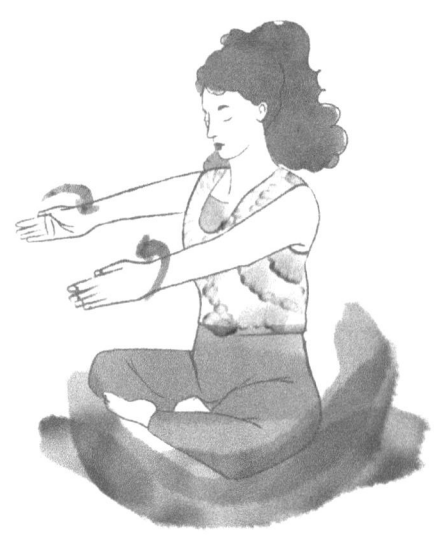
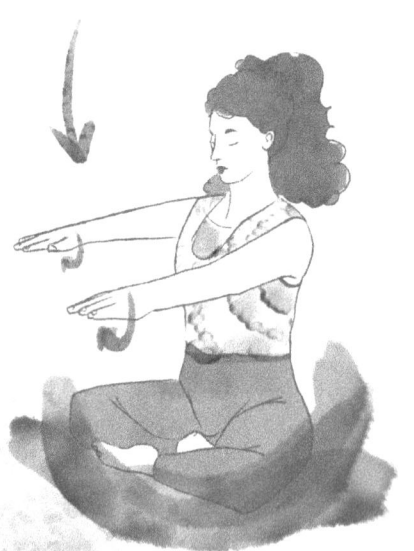

33 / **Resolve Anger for Inner Balance**

March 1, 1999

Sit in Easy Pose with a straight spine and a light Neck Lock.

Mudra: Stretch the arms straight forward parallel to the ground, wider than the shoulders, hands are open and facing each other with fingers relaxed. Rapidly twist the hands from facing each other to facing the ground. Move rapidly, ideally 3 times per second.

Eye Focus: Not specified.

Breath: Not specified.

Time: 3–11 minutes.

To End: Stretch the arms straight up beside the ears and breathe normally in this posture for **30 seconds**.

Comments: Unresolved inner anger from past experiences and insecurities can consume much of our energy. If we instead face these challenges, we can progress. Then we commit to a discipline, whatever it may be. Commitment can balance karma with dharma and give us the capacity to obey, and, as Guru Nanak said, one who obeys shall command the universe. This kriya focuses and balances our internal energy, so instead of passing time and wasting our energy defending the ego, we can commit and face our challenges directly.

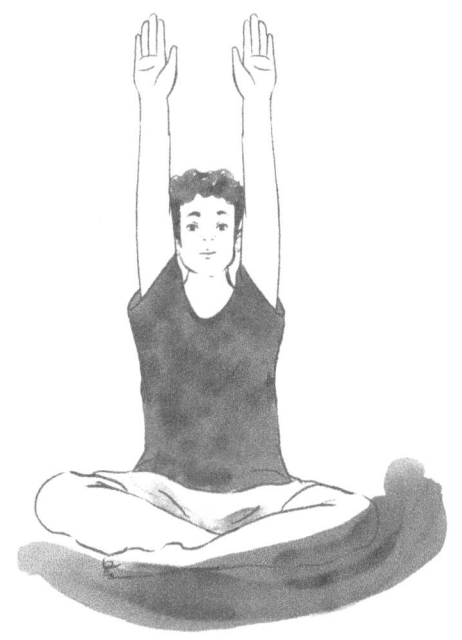

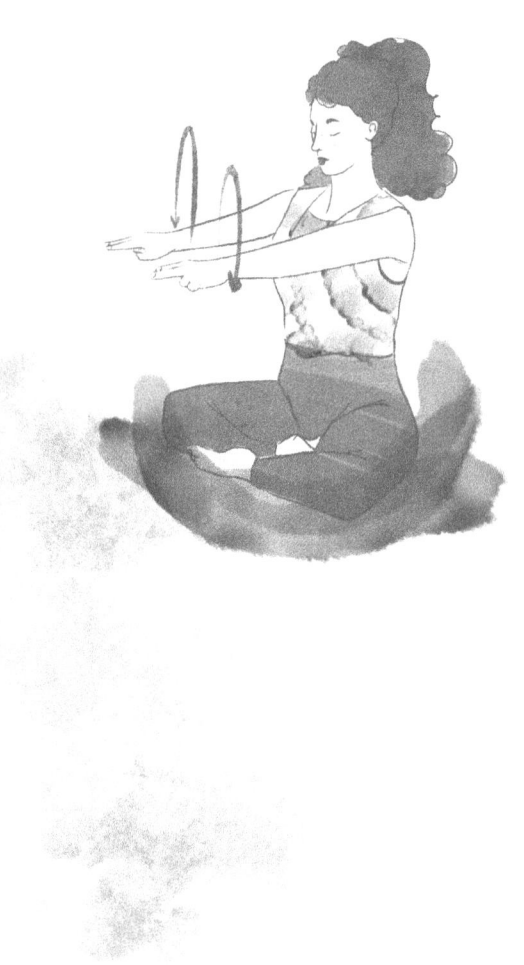

34 / **Let Go of Self-Judgment**

March 2, 1999

Sit in Easy Pose with a straight spine and a light Neck Lock.

Mudra: Extend the Jupiter (index) and Saturn (middle) fingers of both hands and hold the other fingers down with the thumbs. Stretch the arms straight forward with the hands facing down. Rapidly make outward circles from the level of the Arcline (earlobes) to the level of the Heart Center at a pace of 3 times per second.

Eye Focus: Not specified.

Breath: Not specified.

Time: 11 minutes.

To End: Move as quickly as possible for the last minute, inhale, exhale, and relax.

Comments: Inner anger prevents us from relating to and respecting our real selves. In this negative self-judgment, we become insecure and reject our true selves, putting on various masks. The more we hide who we really are, the more habitual it becomes, until we confuse the masks for ourselves. By letting go of self-judgment, we can live authentically.

35 / **Use Shabad to Know Your Impact**

April 12, 1999

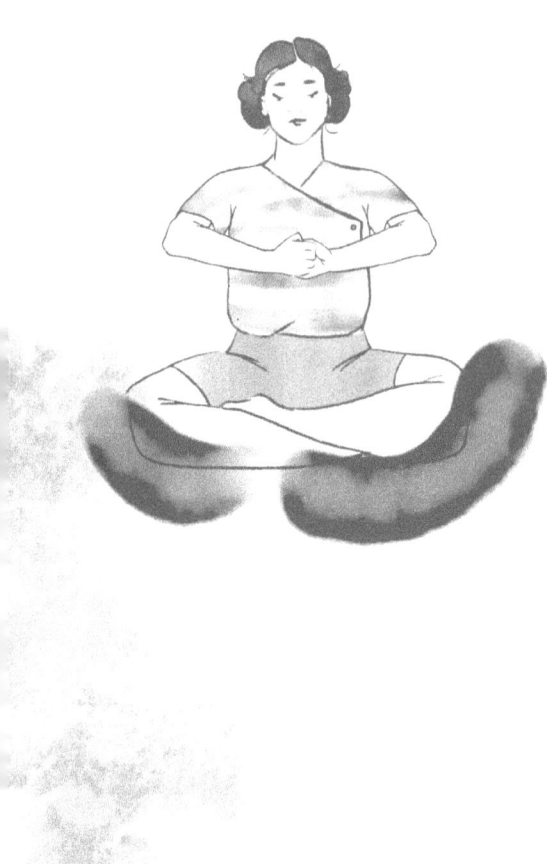

PART ONE
Sit in Easy Pose with a straight spine and a light Neck Lock.

Mudra: Lock the hands in Bear Grip in front of the Heart Center. The left palm faces out and the right palm faces the chest; hook the fingers of the hands together. Keep the forearms parallel to the ground, and pull the lock with maximum strength without releasing it.

Eye Focus: 1/10th open, focused on the Tip of the Nose.

Breath: Not specified.

Mantra: Chant
CHATTR CHAKKR VARTEE.
CHATTR CHAKKR VARTEE,
CHATTR CHAKKR BHUGATAY
SUYUMBHAV SUBHANG
SARAB DAA SARAB JUGTAY
DUKAALANG PRANAASEE
DAYAALANG SAROOPAY
SADAA UNG SUNGAY
ABHANGANG BIBHOOTAY

Time: 9 minutes.

PART TWO
Remain in Easy Pose.

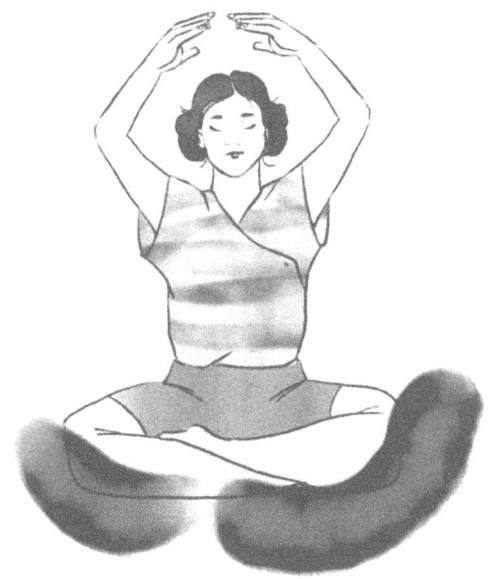

Mudra: Make an arc with the arms on each side of the head, with space between the hands, creating an Adi Shakti with the arms and head.

Eye Focus: Not specified.

Breath: Not specified.

Mantra: Chant the Guru Gaitri mantra with 4 **HARs**.

**HAR HAR HAR HAR
GOBINDAY
HAR HAR HAR HAR
MUKUNDAY
HAR HAR HAR HAR UDAARAY
HAR HAR HAR HAR APAARAY
HAR HAR HAR HAR
HAREEUNG
HAR HAR HAR HAR
KAREEUNG
HAR HAR HAR HAR
NIRNAAMAY
HAR HAR HAR HAR
AKAAMAY**

Time: 3 minutes.

Comments: For the best effect, chant strongly from the navel.

CONTINUE ON NEXT PAGE »

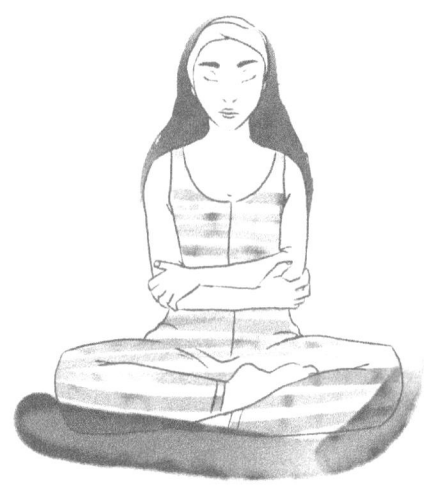

PART THREE
Remain in Easy Pose.

Mudra: Lock the arms with the right hand holding the left arm just above the elbow and the left hand holding the right elbow. Press the arms strongly against the body.

Eye Focus: Not specified.

Breath: Not specified.

Mantra: Chant **KAAL AKAAL** mantra.

**KAAL AKAAL SIREE AKAAL
MAHAA AKAAL
AKAAL MOORAT WHAA-HAY
GUROO**

Time: 3 minutes.

To End: Inhale deeply, suspend the breath for **10 seconds**, squeeze the body, tighten the arm lock, and exhale. Repeat **2 more times**.

Comments: During the Aquarian Age, we need to know the impact and effect of our actions. In this kriya, we experience three shabads to gain this awareness.

36 / Conquer Inner Anger and Burn it Out

March 8, 1999

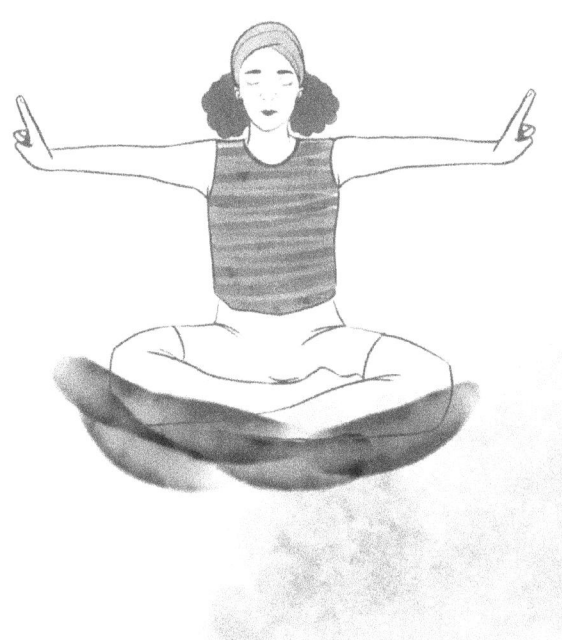

PART ONE
Sit in Easy Pose with a straight spine and a light Neck Lock.

Mudra: Extend the Jupiter (index) fingers and hold the other fingers down with the thumbs. Stretch the arms out to the sides parallel to the ground and bend the wrists with the palms facing outward and the Jupiter fingers pointing up.

Eye Focus: Closed, concentrating on the spine.

Breath: Inhale deeply through the rolled tongue and exhale through the nose, as in Sitali Pranayam.

Time: 11 minutes.

To End: Inhale deeply, suspend the breath for **10 seconds**, stretch the arms out to the sides, and exhale. Repeat **2 more times**.

Comments: Sometimes it will hurt. The more it hurts, the greater the anger; the more anger, the deeper the breath; the deeper we breathe, the less anger we feel.

CONTINUE ON NEXT PAGE »

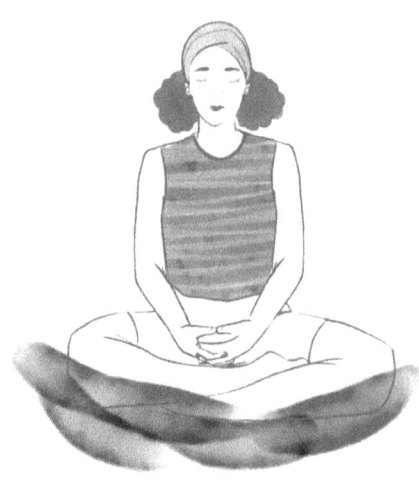

PART TWO
Remain in Easy Pose with a straight spine and a light Neck Lock.

Mudra: Interlace the hands in the lap.

Eye Focus: Closed.

Mantra and Breath:
a) Sing **God and Me, Me and God Are One** for **3 minutes**.
b) do a powerful Breath of Fire for **3 minutes**.
c) Cannon Breath for **1 minute**.

Total Time: 7 minutes.

To End: Inhale deeply, press the hands on the Heart Center, squeeze the body, and suspend the breath for **10 seconds**. Repeat **one more time**. Inhale, suspend the breath, twist the torso to the left, twist to the right, and exhale to the center.

Comments: From birth through childhood, we are frequently under the control of our parents and other people and are unable to express our unique selves. This builds up layers and layers of inner anger until, like a volcano, it erupts. We lose control, and rather than communicating our feelings, we lash out, and our words hurt others. They become afraid, and relationships suffer. The best way around this is to conquer our inner anger and burn it out.

37 / Releasing Childhood Anger

March 9, 1999

Sit in Easy Pose with a straight spine and a light Neck Lock.

Mudra: Extend the Jupiter (index) and Saturn (middle) fingers and hold the other fingers down with the thumbs. Stretch the arms out to the sides parallel to the ground, with the palms facing forward and the fingers together pointing to the sides.

Eye Focus: Not specified.

Breath: Sitkari Breath, also known as hissing breath. Part the lips, with the front teeth gently touching and the tongue resting on the upper palate. Inhale through the teeth, creating a hissing sound. Close the mouth and exhale through the nose.

Time: 11 minutes.

To End: Inhale deeply, suspend the breath for **10 seconds** as you stretch the arms out to the sides, and exhale. Repeat **2 more times.**

Comments: This meditation can awaken subtle powers that change us from within. When this meditation is practiced in the evening, you will notice changes in your energy the next morning.

Childhood anger prevents us from accessing our innate intuition and wisdom. Instead of reacting emotionally to life's challenges, go to your altar and release them to conquer the mind and nurture your relationship with your soul. There, the Divine talks to you.

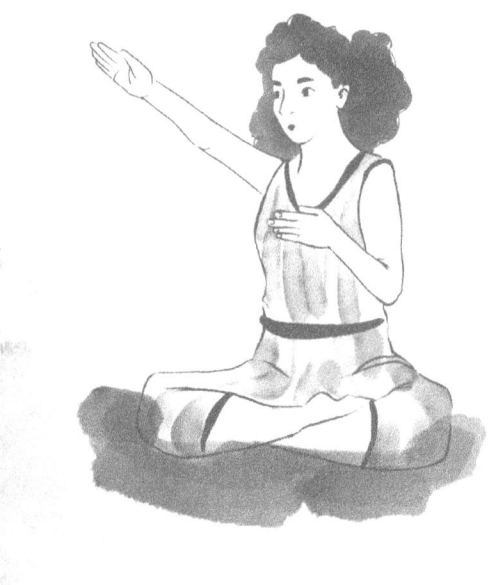

38 / **Trust God To Pave The Way**

April 13, 1999

PART ONE
Sit in Easy Pose with a straight spine and a light Neck Lock.

Mudra: Place the left hand on the Heart Center. Stretch the right arm straight forward and up to a 60-degree angle, with the palm flat and fingers together. There is no bend in the elbow or wrist.

Eye Focus: Open, looking straight ahead.

Breath: Inhale and exhale through puckered lips.

Mantra & Mental Focus: Mentally chant **SAT NAAM** on the inhale and **WHAA-HAY GUROO** on the exhale. Meditate in the name of God.

Time: 2 minutes. Inhale deeply, exhale, and begin Part Two.

Comments: If you practice repeating this mantra mentally, it becomes ingrained in your mind and psyche. Then, when you are stressed, even at the time of death, you will hear the mantra and you will be liberated.

PART TWO
Remain in Easy Pose.

Mudra: Clasp the hands firmly together, palm to palm, with the fingers folded over the back of the opposite hand, in front of the Heart Center. Squeeze the hands tightly.

Eye Focus: Open, looking straight ahead.

Breath: Not specified.

Mantra: Chant **SAT NAAM WHAA-HAY GUROO** once every 3 seconds.

Time: 3 minutes. Inhale deeply, exhale, and begin Part Three.

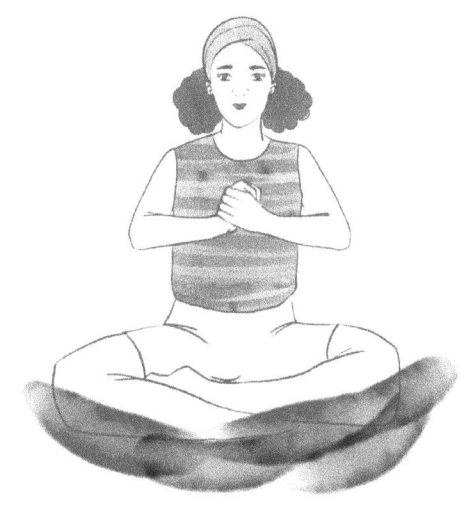

PART THREE
Remain in Easy Pose.

Mudra: Touch the thumbs to the fleshy mound at the base of the Mercury (little) fingers and make fists, folding the fingers over the thumbs. Place the fists in front of the body and rapidly revolve the fists around each other in outward circles.

Eye Focus: Open, looking straight ahead.

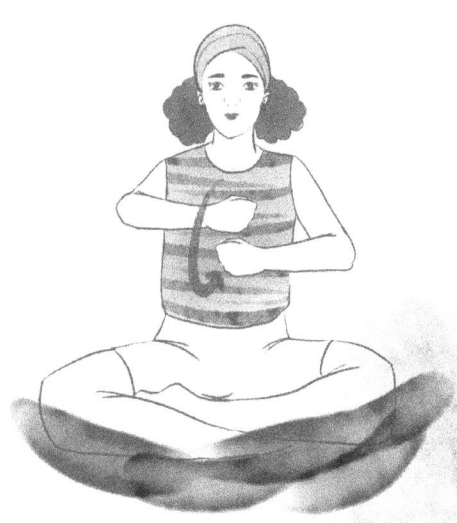

CONTINUE ON NEXT PAGE »

Breath: Not specified.

Mantra: Chant **SAT NAAM WHAA-HAY GUROO** in the same rhythm as Part Two, while the fists rotate rapidly, not in rhythm with the mantra.

Time: 3 minutes.

To End: Inhale deeply, exhale, and begin Part Four.

PART FOUR
Remain in Easy Pose.

Mudra: Place the hands on the Heart Center, right on top of the left.

Eye Focus: Closed.

Breath: Long Deep Breathing.

Mental Focus: Disconnect from the outer world, drop your body, and rise above it so that you can observe yourself from above. Balance the energy and become calm. Feel the love of God in your heart.

Time: 3 minutes.

To End: Inhale deeply, suspend the breath for **15 seconds**, press the hands firmly against the Heart Center, squeeze the body, and distribute the energy to every cell

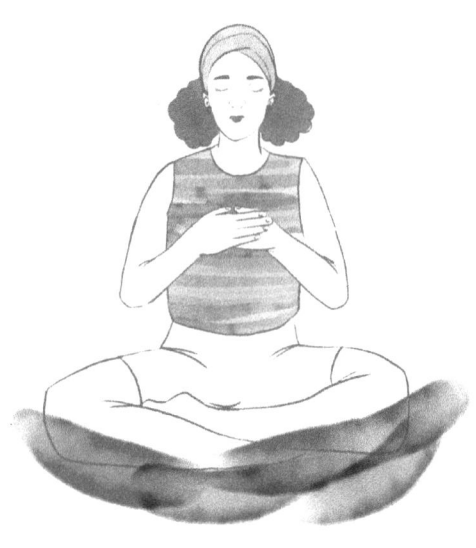

of the body; exhale. Repeat **1 more time.** Inhale deeply, suspend the breath for **15 seconds**, stretch the spine upward, squeeze the body, and distribute the energy to every cell of the body; exhale.

Comments: Because of the ego, we misunderstand and approach life as "I," forgetting about "Thou." When we acknowledge that the Creator is the doer and surrender to this, our trust deepens as God prepares the environment and circumstances we need.

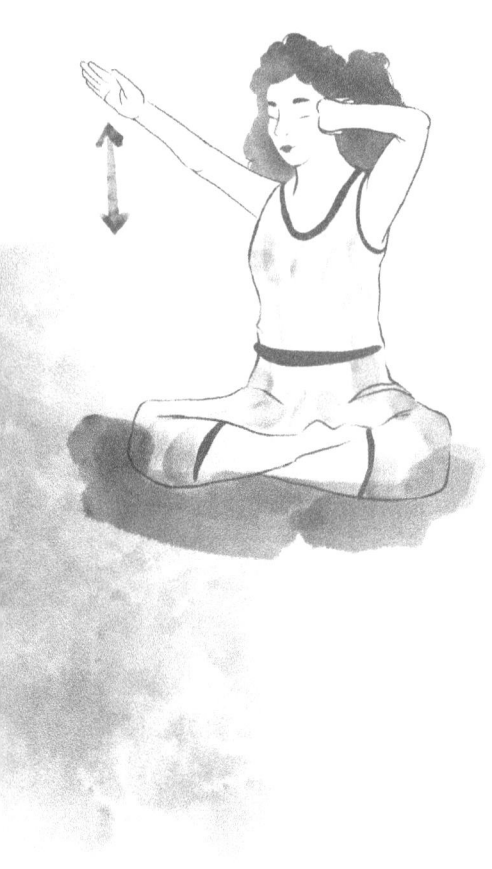

39 / **Experience Interconnectedness**

May 3, 1999

PART ONE
Sit in Easy Pose with a straight spine and a light Neck Lock.

Mudra and Mantra: Press the left palm firmly over the left ear, with the fingers pointing toward the back, pull the elbow back and apply pressure to the ear. Stretch the right arm straight forward and up to a 60-degree angle with the hand facing down and fingers together. Chant **HAR** as you lower the arm 12 inches (30 cm) and chant **HAR** as you raise it back to the starting position.

Eye Focus: Not specified.

Breath: Not specified.

Time: 5 minutes.

To End: Inhale deeply in the starting position and suspend the breath for **15 seconds**. Exhale, and immediately begin Part Two.

PART TWO
Sit in Easy Pose with a straight spine and a light Neck Lock.

Mudra: Remain in the starting position from Part One.

Eye Focus: Not specified.

Breath: Breathe long, slowly, and deeply. Keep a strong pressure on the ear and let the kundalini energy rise.

Time: 3 minutes.

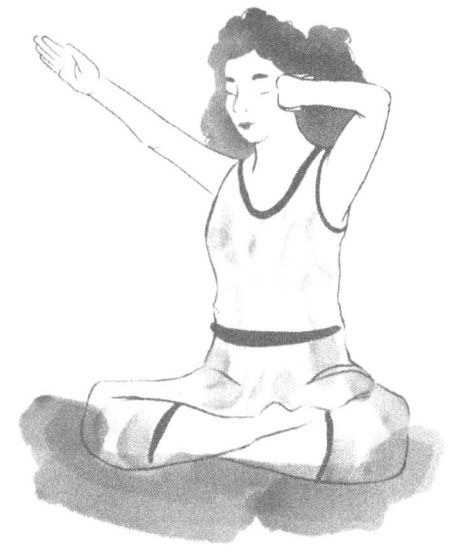

PART THREE
Sit in Easy Pose with a straight spine and a light Neck Lock.

Mudra: Relax the hands down into the lap. Sit very still, calmly, and quietly, and allow the energy to circulate. Meditate deeply, as if you have been meditating for thousands of years.

Eye Focus: Not specified.

Breath: Long Deep Breathing.

Time: 3 minutes.

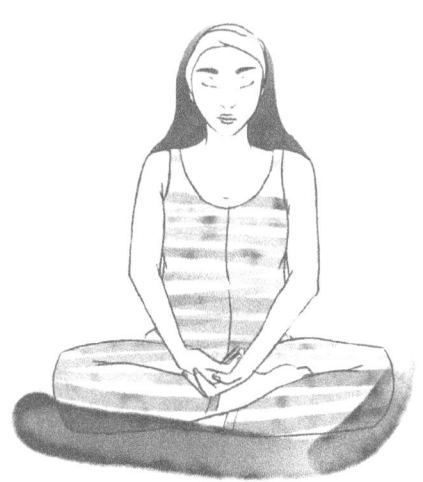

CONTINUE ON NEXT PAGE »

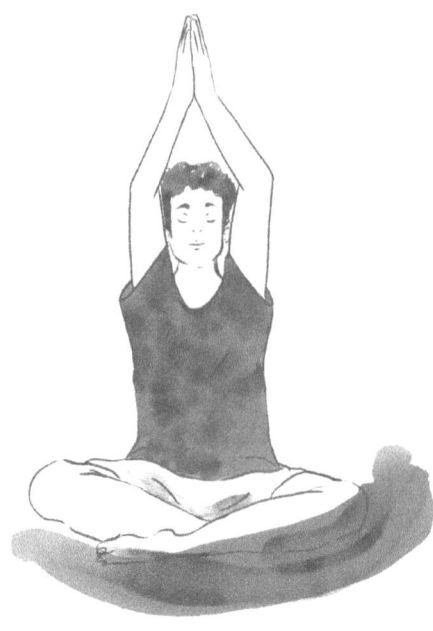

PART FOUR
Remain in Easy Pose with a straight spine and a light Neck Lock.

Mudra: Stretch the arms straight up with the hands in Prayer Pose.

Eye Focus: Not specified.

Breath: Long Deep Breathing.

Time: 2 minutes.

To End: Inhale deeply, suspend the breath for **15 seconds**, and Cannon Fire exhale. Relax and talk to someone for **5 minutes**. (If practicing alone, talk to yourself.)

Comments: This posture is self-healing.

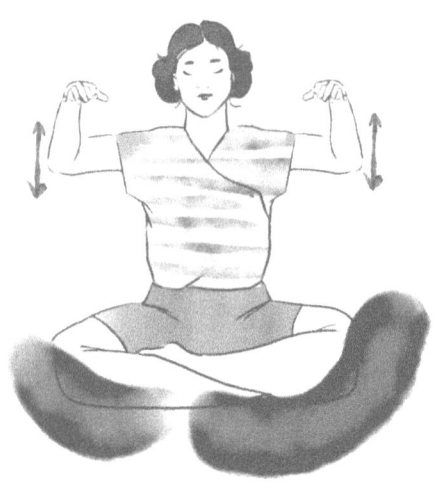

PART FIVE
Sit in Easy Pose with a straight spine and a light Neck Lock.

Mudra: Bend the elbows at shoulder level, bring the arms out to the sides, and bring the forearms forward and angled up. The wrists are bent and the hands relaxed. Rapidly, rhythmically, raise and lower the shoulders, bouncing the arms and hands up and down a few inches (8–10 cm).

Eye Focus: Closed.

Breath: Breath of Fire.

Time: 11 minutes.

To End: Inhale deeply, exhale, and immediately begin Part Six.

PART SIX
Remain in Easy Pose.

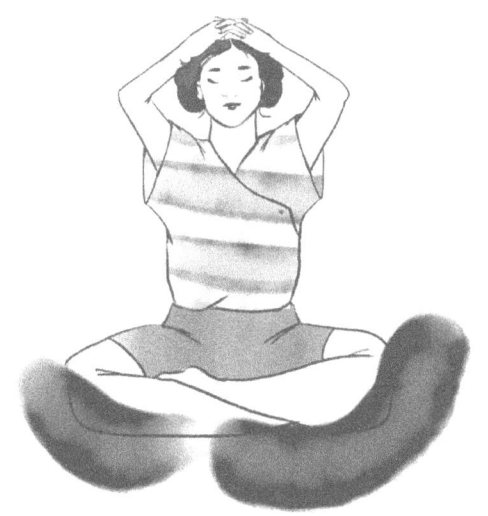

Mudra: Interlace the fingers and place them on top of the head, with elbows out to the sides. Rest the weight of the hands on the head.

Eye Focus: Not specified.

Breath: Long Deep Breathing.

Mantra:
a) Listen to a recording of the mantra **GUROO GUROO, WHAA-HAY GUROO, GUROO RAM DAS GUROO** for **13 minutes**.
b) Chant **RAKHAY RAKHANHAAR** from the navel for **8 minutes**. (The recording by Singh Kaur was played in the original class.)

**RAKHAY RAKHANHAAR AAP UBAARIUN
GUR KEE PAIREE PAA-EH
KAAJ SAVAARIUN
HOAA AAP DAYAAL MANHO**

CONTINUE ON NEXT PAGE »

NA VISAARIUN
SAADH JANAA KAI SUNG
BHAVJAL TAARIUN
SAAKAT NINDAK DUSHT
KHIN MAA-EH BIDAARIUN
TIS SAAHIB KEE TAYK
NAANAK MANAI MAA-EH
JIS SIMRAT SUKH HO-EH
SAGLAY DOOKH JAA-EH

c) Strongly whisper **RAKHAY RAKHANHAAR** for **4 minutes**.
d) Listen to the recording of **RAKHAY RAKHANHAAR** for the last **1 minute**.

Total Time: 26 minutes.

To End: Inhale deeply, suspend the breath for **15 seconds**, stretch the spine, and press down on top of the head. Exhale. Repeat **2 more times**.

Comments: In the Aquarian Age, human beings will operate from their senses of spirituality and interconnectedness. Each person's wholeness, or internal balance, will communicate with another's. Experience interconnectedness in this kriya so you can heal, hold space for deep emotions, and share love.

40 / Use Your Energy to Live Your Own Truth

May 4, 1999

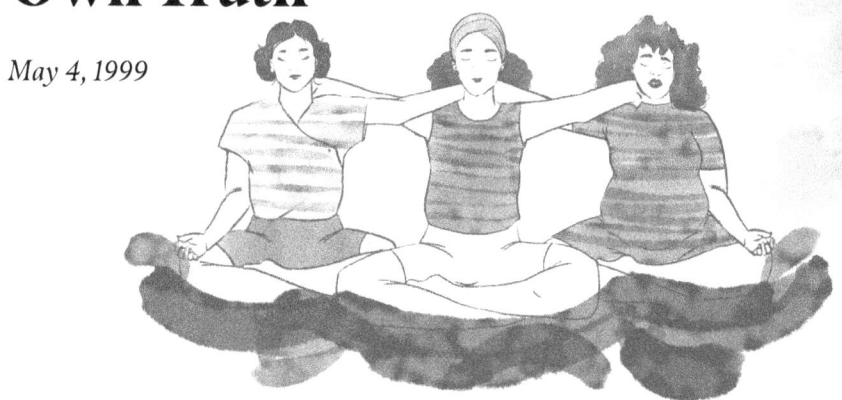

In a class or group situation, each person sits near others in Easy Pose with a straight spine and a light Neck Lock.

Mudra: Grasp the back of the neck of the people seated on either side of you. (If you are on the end, grasp with one hand and relax the other hand in the lap.)

Eye Focus: 1/10th open focused on the Tip of the Nose.

Breath: Not specified.

Mantra: a) Chant from the navel the Siri Gaitri Mantra: **RAA MAA DAA SAA, SAA SAY SO HUNG** for **38 minutes**.
b) Whisper powerfully for **1 minute**.
c) Stick the tongue out as far as you can for **1 minute**.

Total Time: 40 minutes.

To End: Inhale deeply, suspend the breath for **15 seconds**, squeeze the spine and body, and Cannon Fire exhale. Repeat **2 more times**.

Comments: We can waste energy living for others, trying to please others. We can feel pressure to conform to the way our ancestors lived and suffer guilt when we make different choices. We can lie and hide our insecurities under many layers, but if our higher Selves are integrated within us, we do not waver. When we know our own purity and God within us, we can be fully ourselves and live our own truth.

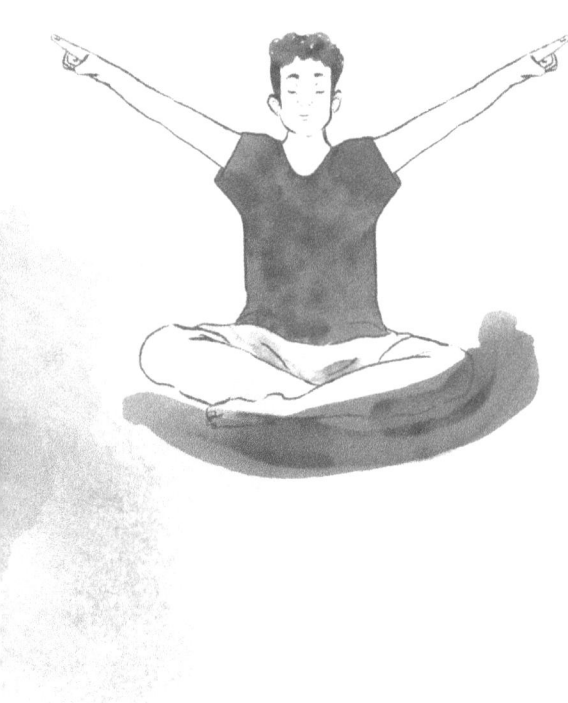

41 / Become Vast and Open to Everything

May 5, 1999

Sit in Easy Pose with a straight spine and a light Neck Lock.

Mudra: Extend the Jupiter (index) fingers of both hands and hold the other fingers down with the thumbs. Raise the arms up 60 degrees from parallel and out 60 degrees from center. Stretch out from the shoulders.

Eye Focus: 1/10th open, looking at the Tip of the Nose.

Breath and Mantra: a) Cannon Breath for **3–11 minutes.** b) Chant **WHAA-HAY GUROO, WHAA-HAY GUROO, WHAA-HAY GUROO, WHAA-HAY JEEO** for **3–11 minutes.** (The recording "Wahe Guru, Wahe Guru, Wahe Guru, Wahe Jio" by Gyani Ji was played in the original class.) c) Whisper the mantra for **3–11 minutes.**

Total Time: 9–33 minutes.

To End: Inhale deeply, suspend the breath for **10 seconds**, stretch the spine and arms, and Cannon Fire exhale. Repeat **2 more times**. Stretch and massage your arms and shoulders.

Comments: When our mind is ruled by the ego, our life is small and limited, and we miss opportunities. When we clear our subconscious, life is vast and limitless.

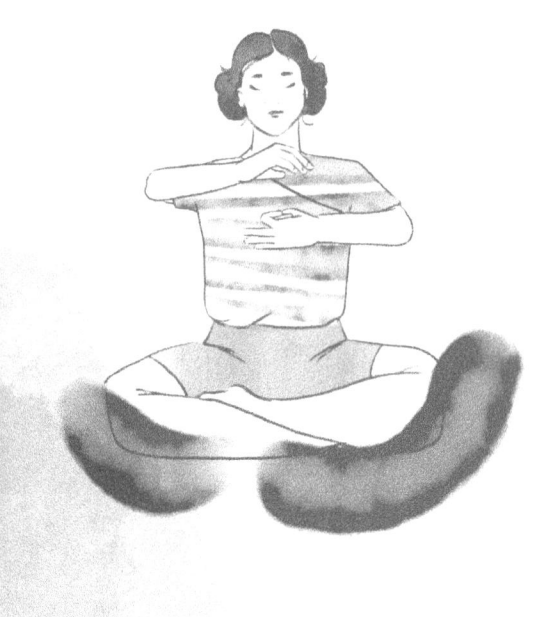

42 / **Kriya To Reveal the Core Reality of You**

May 13, 1999

PART ONE
Sit in Easy Pose with a straight spine and a light Neck Lock.

Mudra: Place the left hand in front of the Heart Center with the palm facing the body. Create a circle with the tips of the thumb and Jupiter (index) finger touching and the other three fingers relaxed. Place the right hand above the circle at the level of the Throat Center, facing down, and curved to form a dome, as if you are passing light from the right hand through the hole of the left hand. The elbows are out to the sides, with both forearms parallel to the ground.

Eye Focus: 1/10th open, focused on the Tip of the Nose.

Breath: Long Deep Breathing.

Time: 15 minutes. Immediately begin Part Two.

PART TWO
Remain in Easy Pose.

Mudra: Relax the elbows at the sides of the body and bring the hands up facing the body with the tips of the Mercury (little) fingers and the side of the base of the palms touching. There is space between the sides of the cupped hands, and they are held in front of the Heart Center.

Eye Focus: 1/10th open, focused on the Tip of the Nose.

Breath: Long Deep Breathing.

Time: 3 minutes. Immediately begin Part Three.

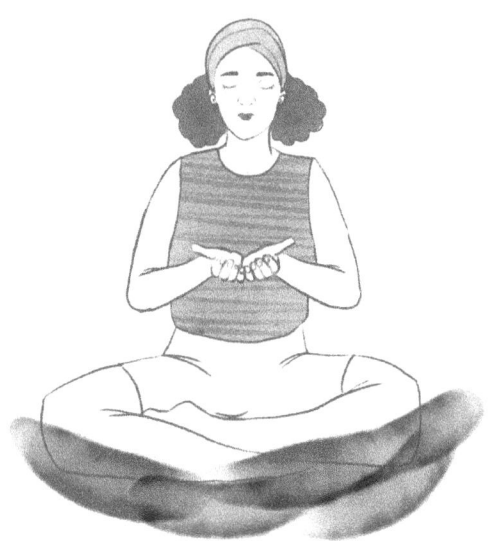

PART THREE
Remain in Easy Pose.

Mudra: Stretch the arms straight forward from the shoulders parallel to the ground with the hands facing down and fingers separated wide and stiff. Keep the fingers straight and firm.

Eye Focus: 1/10th open, focused on the Tip of the Nose.

Breath: Long Deep Breathing.

Mental Focus: Allow the energy of the universe to come in through the fingers and flow throughout the body.

Time: 9 minutes.

CONTINUE ON NEXT PAGE »

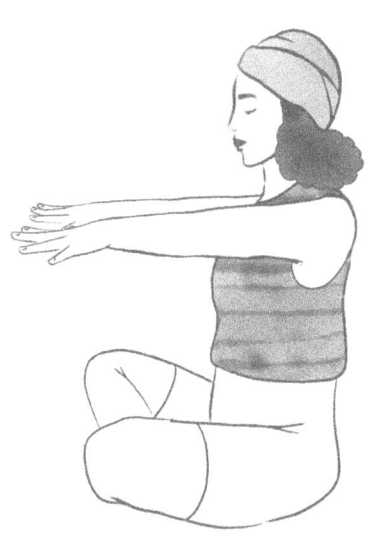

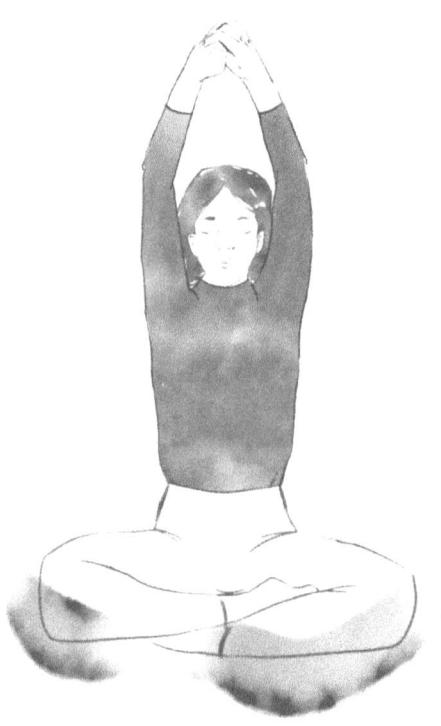

To End: Interlace the fingers in Venus Lock and stretch the arms up strongly. Inhale deeply, suspend the breath for 10 seconds, and exhale. Repeat **2 more times.**

Comments: You may play light, uplifting Kundalini music to support the practice. (An unpublished recording of the Triple Mantra by Joseph Michael Levry was played in the original class.) Work with the Pavan Guru, the breath of life, in this kriya to affect the psyche and change our mental projection. Relax the body by slowing the breath, and go deeply within. Our faculties will grow, bring prosperity, and reveal our simple core reality.

breathe, rest, concentrate

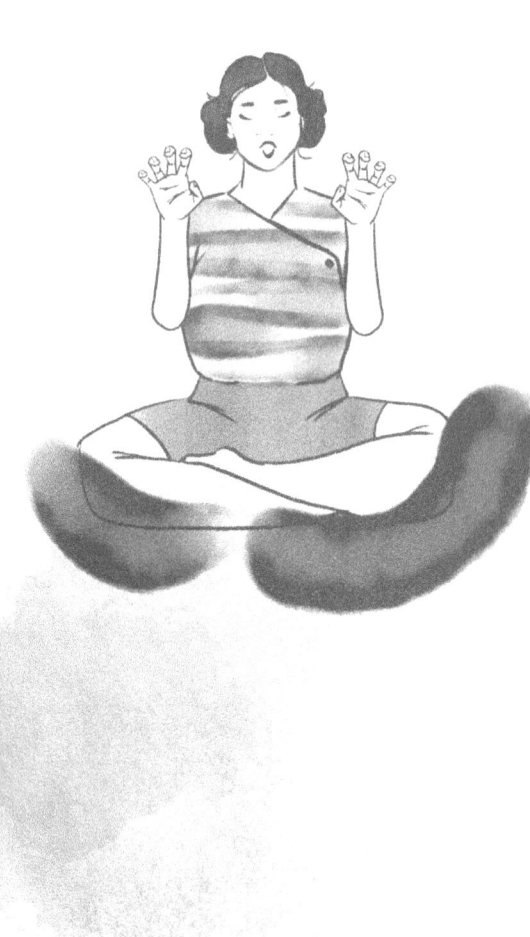

43 / **Expand Into Your Excellence**

May 14, 1999

PART ONE
Sit in Easy Pose with a straight spine and a light Neck Lock.

Mudra: Rest the elbows at the sides, make claws of your hands with the forearms perpendicular to the ground and bring them by the shoulders with the palms facing forward.

Eye Focus: Not specified.

Breath: Cannon Breath.

Mantra: You can listen to a mantra to uplift you. (The recording "Triple Mantra" by Dr. Joseph Michael Levry was played in the original class.)

Time: 2 ½ minutes.

To End: Inhale deeply and immediately begin Part Two.

PART TWO
Remain in Easy Pose.

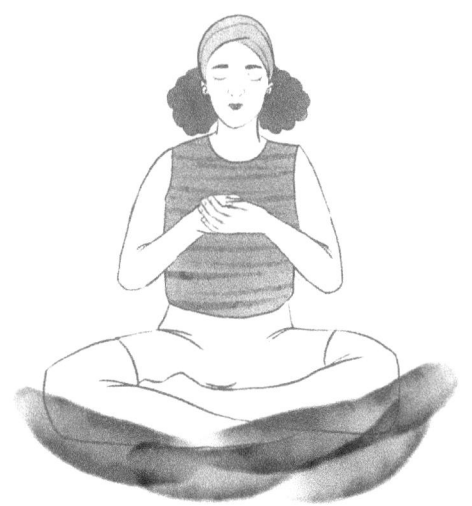

Mudra & Breath: Make a fist of the right hand in front of the Heart Center, palm facing the body. Place the left hand on top of the fist. Inhale deeply, suspend the breath for as long as possible, press down with the left hand and resist with the fist, then exhale.

Eye Focus: Not specified.

Mantra: You can listen to a mantra to uplift you. (The recording "Triple Mantra" by Dr. Joseph Michael Levry was played in the original class.)

Time: 5 minutes.

To End: Inhale deeply, exhale, and immediately begin Part Three.

PART THREE
Remain in Easy Pose.

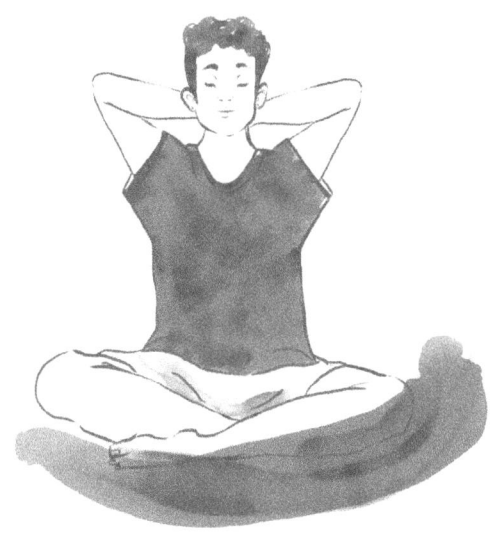

Mudra: Interlace the fingers on the back of the neck with the elbows stretched out to the sides. Press with the hands and resist with the neck.

Eye Focus: Not specified.

Breath: Not specified.

CONTINUE ON NEXT PAGE »

Mantra: Chant the Triple Mantra from the navel. (The recording by Dr. Joseph Michael Levry was played in the original class.)

**AAD GURAY NAMEH
JUGAAD GURAY NAMEH
SATGURAY NAMEH
SIREE GURDAYV-AY NAMEH
AAD SUCH JUGAAD SUCH
HAIBHEE SUCH
NAANAK HOSEE BHEE SUCH
AAD SUCH JUGAAD SUCH
HAIBHEI SUCH
NAANAK HOSEE BHEI SUCH**

Time: 4 ½ minutes.

To End: Inhale deeply, suspend the breath for **10 seconds**, maintain tension between the hands and the neck, stretch the spine up, and Cannon Fire exhale. Repeat **2 more times.**

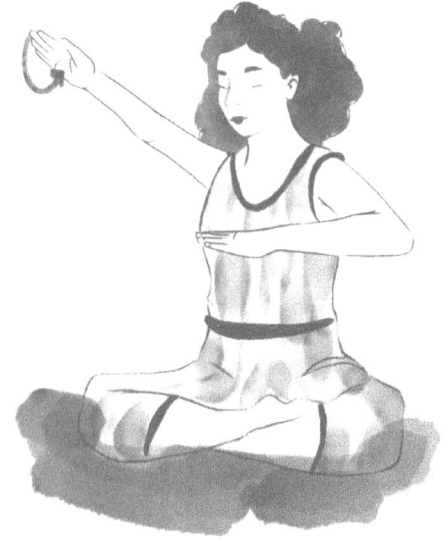

PART FOUR
Sit in Easy Pose with a straight spine and a light Neck Lock.

Mudra and Mantra: Bring the left forearm parallel to the ground with the hand in front of the Heart Center, palm facing down. Bring the right arm straight forward and up to a 60-degree angle, palm facing down with the fingers together. Keep the right elbow and wrist straight. Listen to a recording of Jaap Sahib and bend the right fingers to the base of the palm with each repetition of "Namastang" or "Namo". Without the recording, the movement is done to 10 beats as follows: bend them in 2 counts for 4 cycles, and rest in the starting position on counts 9 and 10. (The recording "Jaap Sahib" by Satnam Singh Sethi was played in the original class.)

Eye Focus: Not specified.

Breath: Not specified.

Time: 5 minutes.

To End: Inhale deeply, suspend the breath for **15 seconds**, bend the fingers down strongly, and exhale. Inhale deeply, suspend the breath for **10 seconds**, keep the fingers bent tightly, and exhale. Immediately begin Part Five.

PART FIVE
Remain in Easy Pose.

Mudra: Cross the arms in front of the chest and hold onto the opposite shoulders.

Eye Focus: Closed.

CONTINUE ON NEXT PAGE »

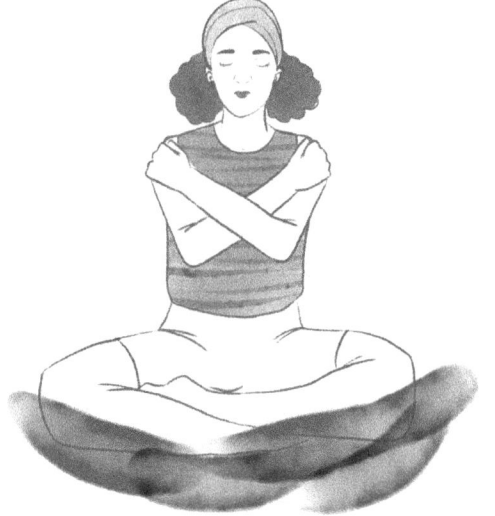

BE YOU

Breath: Not specified.

Mantra: Chant the Guru Gaitri mantra with 4 **HARs** from the navel. (The recording by Nirinjan Kaur, from *White Tantra Volume 1*, was played in the original class.)

**HAR HAR HAR HAR GOBINDAY
HAR HAR HAR HAR MUKUNDAY
HAR HAR HAR HAR UDAARAY
HAR HAR HAR HAR APAARAY
HAR HAR HAR HAR HAREEUNG
HAR HAR HAR HAR KAREEUNG
HAR HAR HAR HAR NIRNAAMAY
HAR HAR HAR HAR AKAAMAY**

Time: 10 minutes.

To End: Inhale deeply, suspend the breath for **20 seconds**, press the shoulders inward, and exhale. Repeat **2 more times**, suspending the breath for **10 seconds**.

PART SIX
Remain in Easy Pose.

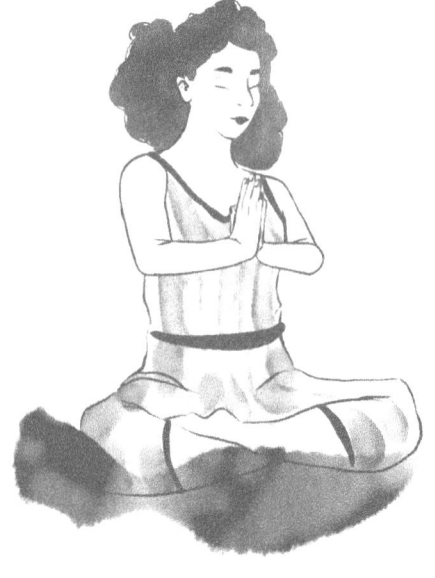

Mudra: Place the hands in Prayer Pose.

Eye Focus: Closed.

Breath: Not specified.

Mental Focus: Mentally repeat the following affirmation: "I am wonderful. I am excellent. I am divine. I am the pure creation of God."

Time: 3 minutes.

Comments: We have the capacity to become elegant, self-sufficient, and creative people. Self-discipline is all that we need to live in an excellent way. We do not need any help from outside. Once we have identified and incorporated our true selves, we can authentically communicate our own opinions, the union of our minds and spirits, simply and gracefully.

44 / **Naad Sutra Kriya**

May 17, 1999

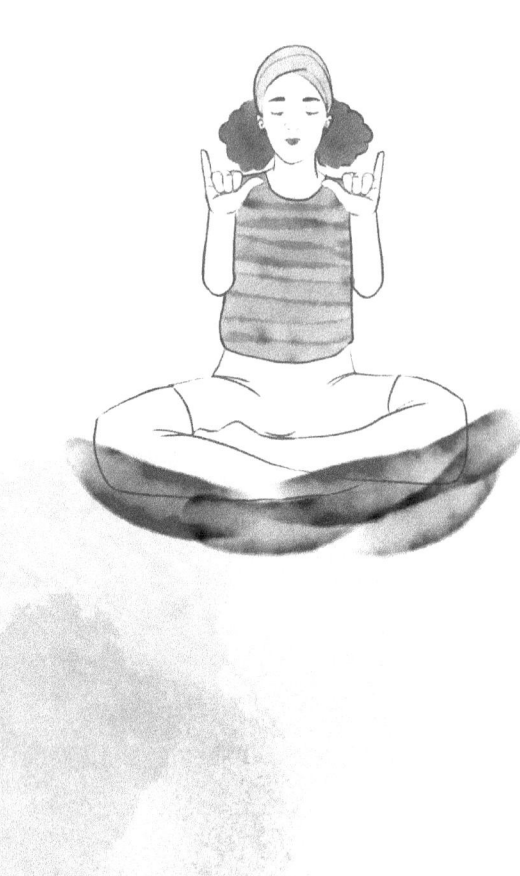

Sit in Easy Pose with a straight spine and a light Neck Lock.

Mudra: Bring the hands by the shoulders, forearms perpendicular to the ground and palms facing forward. Make fists with both hands and extend the thumbs and Mercury (little) fingers.

Eye Focus: Tip of the Nose.

Breath:
a) Not specified for **11 ½ minutes**.
b) Long Deep Breathing through the "O" mouth for **8 minutes**.
c) Cannon Breath for **7 minutes**.

Mental Focus: Mentally chant **WHAA-HAY GUROO**.

Mantra: Listen to a recording of the Triple Mantra. (The recording "Triple Mantra" by Dr. Joseph Michael Levry was played in the original class.)

AAD GURAY NAMEH
JUGAAD GURAY NAMEH SAT
GURAY NAMEH
SIREE GURDAYV-AY NAMEH
AAD SUCH JUGAAD SUCH
HAIBHEE SUCH
NAANAK HOSEE BHEE SUCH
AAD SUCH JUGAAD SUCH
HAIBHEI SUCH
NAANAK HOSEE BHEI SUCH
Total Time: 26 ½ minutes.

To End: Inhale deeply, suspend the breath for **10 seconds**, move the diaphragm powerfully, and exhale. Inhale deeply, suspend the breath for **20 seconds**, move the diaphragm, and exhale. Inhale deeply, suspend the breath for **20 seconds**, move the diaphragm, and exhale.

Comments: Meditating every day cleans our subconscious mind. If the subconscious load becomes too great, it spills into the conscious mind, and the psyche cannot connect the two hemispheres of the brain to effectively process thoughts and act consciously. We meditate for mental hygiene and to remain harmonious, uplifted human beings.

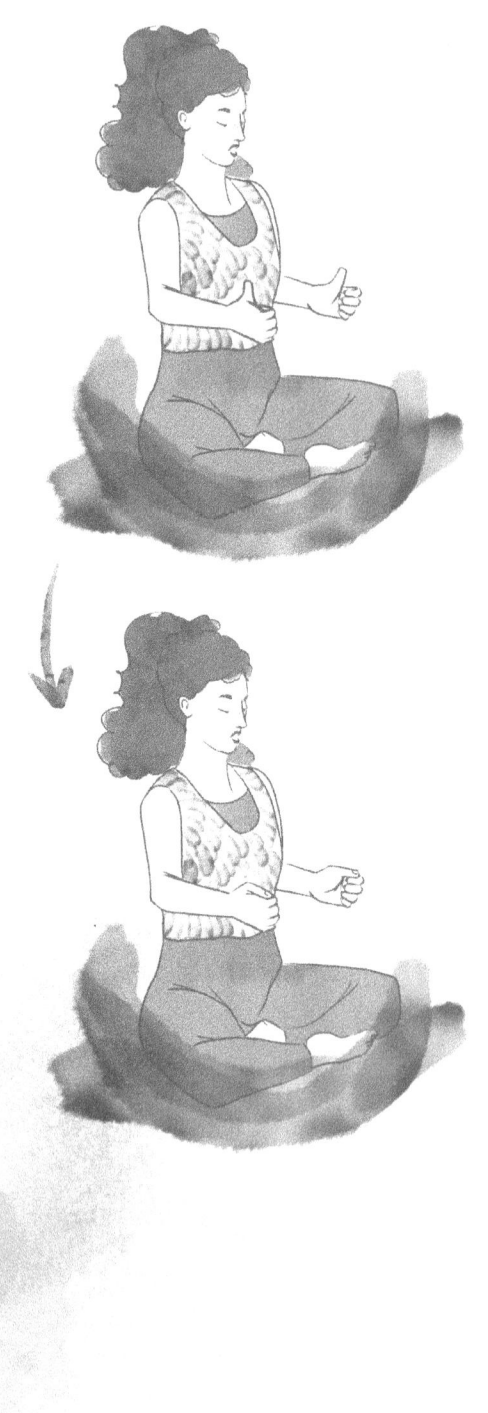

45 / **To Act From the Vastness of Your Heart**

May 18, 1999

PART ONE
Sit in Easy Pose with a straight spine and a light Neck Lock.

Mudra: Relax the elbows next to the body and stretch the forearms forward with the hands in fists and thumbs stretched up. On the inhale, bend the thumbs down on top of the fists. On the exhale, the thumbs return to the starting position.

Eye Focus: Tip of the Nose.

Breath: Powerfully inhale and exhale through the "O" mouth as fast as possible.

Mantra: Listen to the Siri Gaitri Mantra **RAA MAA DAA SAA, SAA SAY SO HUNG.** (Slow and regular versions by Joseph Michael Levry were played in the original class.)

Time: 20 minutes. Immediately begin Part Two.

PART TWO
Remain in Easy Pose.

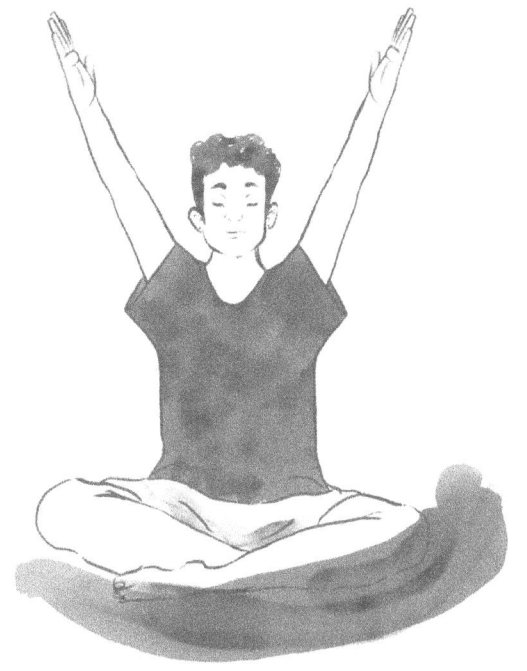

Mudra: Stretch the arms out to the sides and raise them up 60 degrees from horizontal with no bend in the wrist and elbow. Palms are facing up.

Eye Focus: Closed.

Breath & Mantra: Chant the Siri Gaitri Mantra **RAA MAA DAA SAA, SAA SAY SO HUNG.** (The recording by Joseph Michael Levry was played in the original class.)

Time: 3 minutes.

To End: Inhale deeply, maintain the posture with arms stiff, stretch them out from the shoulders, suspend the breath for **20 seconds**, and exhale. Repeat **2 more times**, suspending the breath for **10 seconds**.

Comments: Trust is built through our actions. The mind and the ego are not involved. When we act through intuition from the vastness of our Heart Centers, every action is correct and serves the highest good of all.

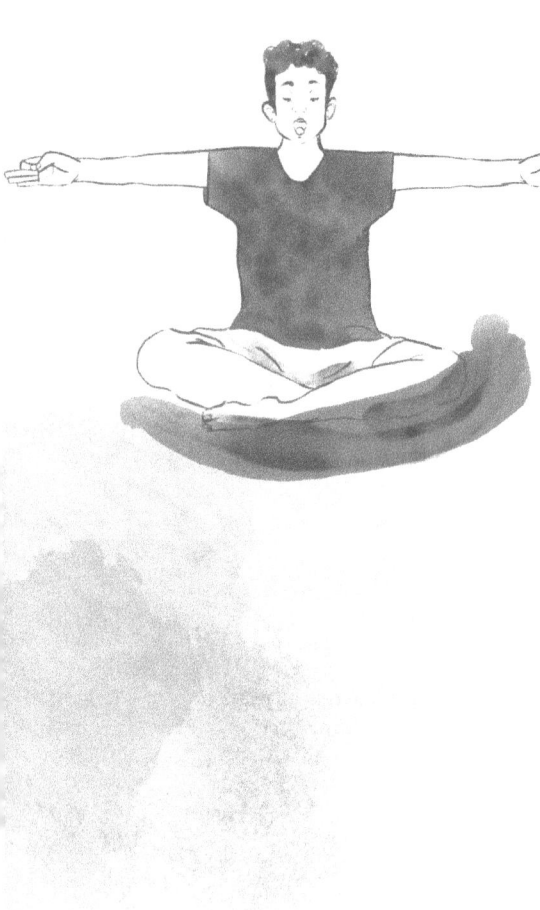

46 / Kriya to Awaken Intuition

May 19, 1999

There are no breaks between the exercises.

PART ONE
Sit in Easy Pose with a straight spine and a light Neck Lock.

Mudra: Touch the tip of the thumbs and the Jupiter (index) fingers in Gyan Mudra. Extend the arms out to the sides parallel to the ground, with the hands facing forward.

Eye Focus: Tip of the Nose.

Breath: Cannon Breath, focusing on powerfully moving the diaphragm. (In the original class, the recording "Tantric Har" by Simran Kaur and Guru Prem Singh was played to keep the rhythm.)

Time: 4 minutes.

PART TWO
Remain in Easy Pose.

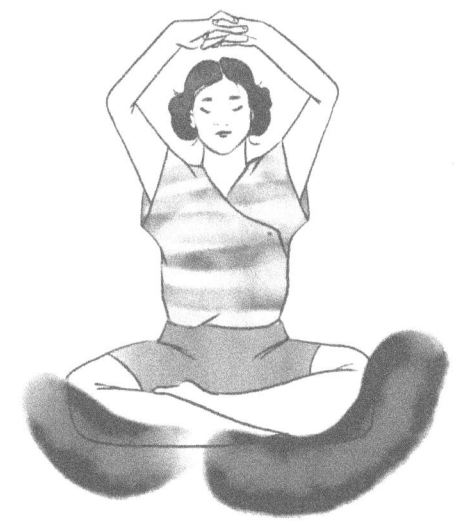

Mudra: Interlace the fingers and raise the arms to form an arc over the head with the palms facing down.

Eye Focus: Tip of the Nose.

Breath: Cannon Breath, focusing on powerfully moving the diaphragm. (In the original class, the recording "Tantric Har" by Simran Kaur and Guru Prem Singh was played to keep the rhythm.)

Time: 2 minutes.

PART THREE
Remain in Easy Pose.

Mudra: Interlace the fingers and place them behind the neck. Stretch the elbows out to the sides with the forearms parallel to the ground. Apply pressure with the hands on the neck and resist with the neck.

Eye Focus: Closed.

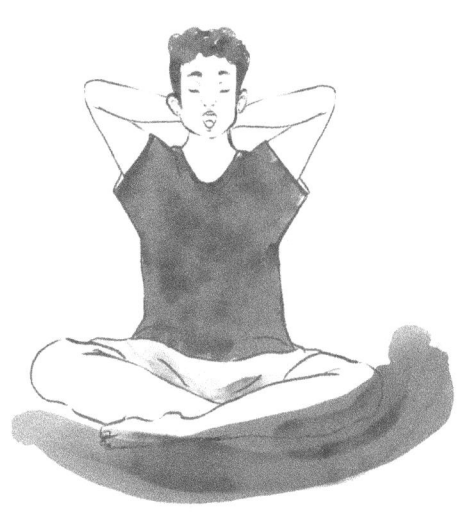

Breath: Cannon Breath, focusing on powerfully moving the diaphragm for **1 minute**. Long Deep Breathing for **5 ½ minutes**.

CONTINUE ON NEXT PAGE »

Total Time: 6 ½ minutes.

To End: Inhale deeply, suspend the breath for **10 seconds**, and move the diaphragm as fast as you can. Exhale. Repeat **2 more times**.

PART FOUR
Remain in Easy Pose.

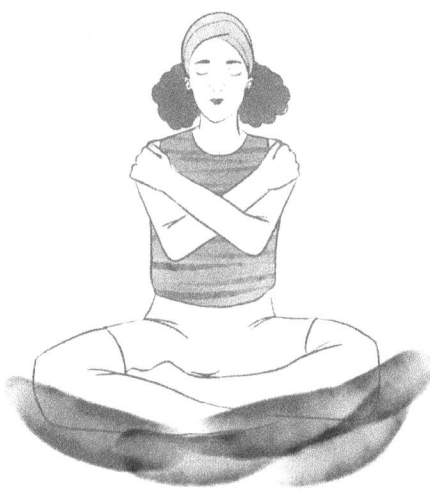

Mudra: Cross the arms on the chest, right arm on top of the left, with hands holding just below the opposite shoulder.

Eye Focus: Closed.

Breath: Not specified.

Visualization: Become thoughtless and travel through the Universe, flying through space and the planes of existence, flying higher and higher beyond the sky, reaching the heavens. Reach higher, elevate yourself, and feel lighter and lighter.

Time: 3 ½ minutes.

To End: Inhale deeply, suspend the breath for **10 seconds**, squeeze the body as strongly as possible, and exhale. Repeat **2 more times**.

Comments: It is recommended to drink plenty of water after practicing this kriya to assist in eliminating toxins released through the postures and powerful movement of the diaphragm. Adding lemon or vitamin C to the water will enhance the elimination process. The animal nature in us is impulsive; by elevating ourselves, we can awaken our divine nature and operate intuitively.

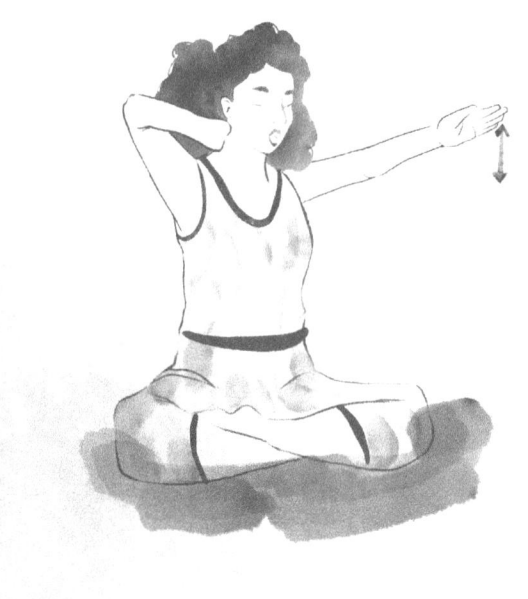

47 / Kriya To Increase Circulation and Energize The Brain

May 20, 1999

PART ONE
Sit in Easy Pose with a straight spine and a light Neck Lock.

Mudra: Place the left hand behind the neck and press the neck. Extend the right arm straight forward, 20 degrees above parallel to the ground, palm facing down. Move the right hand up and down 6 inches (15 cm), keeping the arm straight.

Eye Focus: Not specified.

Breath: Cannon Breath.

Time: 3 minutes. Immediately begin Part Two.

PART TWO
Remain in Easy Pose.

Mudra: Switch the arm positions by placing the right hand behind the neck

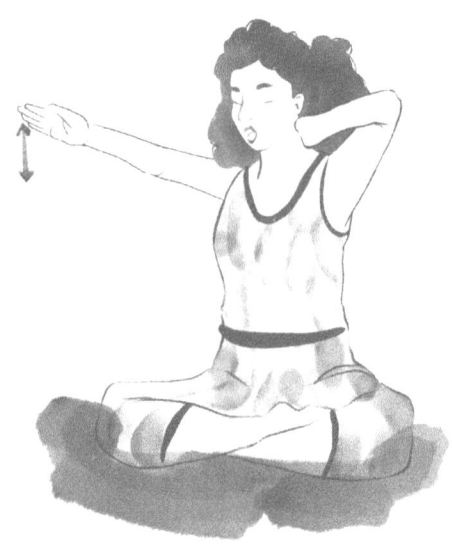

and press. Extend the left arm straight forward, 20 degrees above parallel to the ground, palm facing down. Move the left hand up and down 6 inches (15 cm) with no bend in the elbow.

Eye Focus: Not specified.

Breath: Cannon Breath.

3 minutes. Immediately begin Part Three.

PART THREE
Remain in Easy Pose.

Mudra: Interlace the hands and raise the arms straight up. Twist powerfully from side to side.

Eye Focus: Not specified.

Breath: Cannon Breath.

Time: 3 minutes.

To End: Inhale deeply, suspend the breath for **10 seconds**, and continue the movement. Exhale. Repeat **2 more times**.

Comments: This kriya works on the circulatory system and nourishes the nervous system. You may experience discomfort in the arm, shoulders, or neck as blood rushes to those areas. The powerful Cannon Breath helps to release the diaphragm, bringing increased oxygen into the body. The movement in the final exercise pushes the spinal fluid upward to energize the brain.

BE YOU

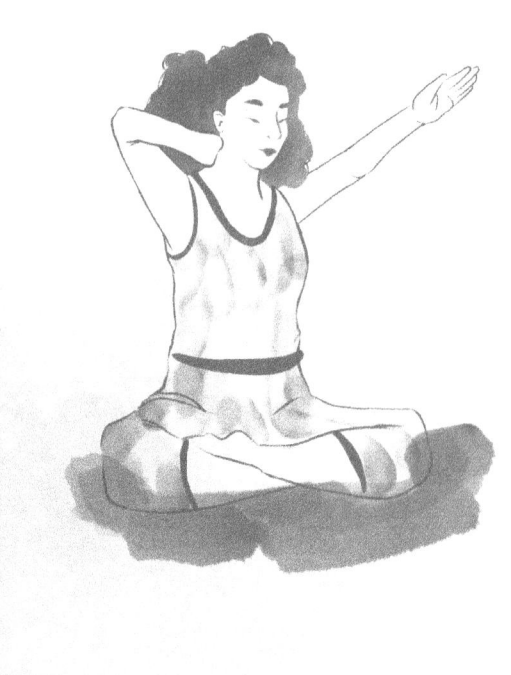

48 / **Kriya to Develop Grit and Grace**

May 24, 1999

PART ONE
Sit in Easy Pose with a straight spine and a light Neck Lock.

Mudra: Place the left hand on the neck and apply forward pressure while resisting with the neck. Extend the right arm forward at a 60-degree angle above parallel and slightly angled out, palm facing down.

Eye Focus: Tip of the Nose.

Breath: Long Deep Breathing.

Mantra: WHAA-HAY GUROO, WHAA-HAY GUROO, WHAA-HAY GUROO, WHAA-HAY JEEO. Pump the navel in rhythm with the music. (Sangeet Kaur and Harjinder Singh's version, from the album *Raga Sadhana* was played in the original class.)

Time: 17 minutes. Immediately begin Part Two.

PART TWO
Remain in Easy Pose.

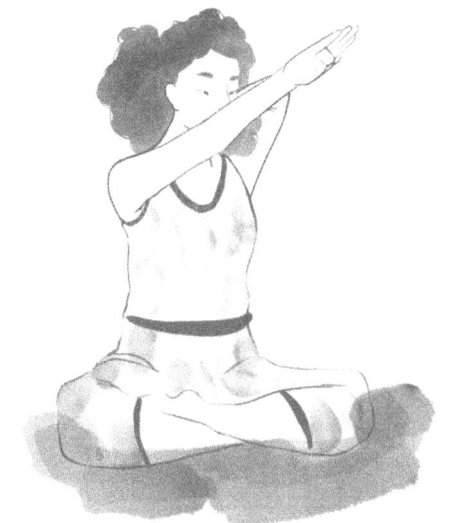

Mudra: Switch arms by placing the right hand behind the neck and applying forward pressure while resisting with the neck. Extend the left arm forward at a 60-degree angle above parallel and slightly angled out, palm facing down.

Eye Focus: Tip of the Nose.

Breath: Long Deep Breathing.

Mantra: WHAA-HAY GUROO, WHAA-HAY GUROO, WHAA-HAY GUROO, WHAA-HAY JEEO. Pump the navel in rhythm with the music. (Sangeet Kaur and Harjinder Singh's version, from the album *Raga Sadhana* was played in the original class.)

Time: 4 ½ minutes. Immediately begin Part Three.

CONTINUE ON NEXT PAGE »

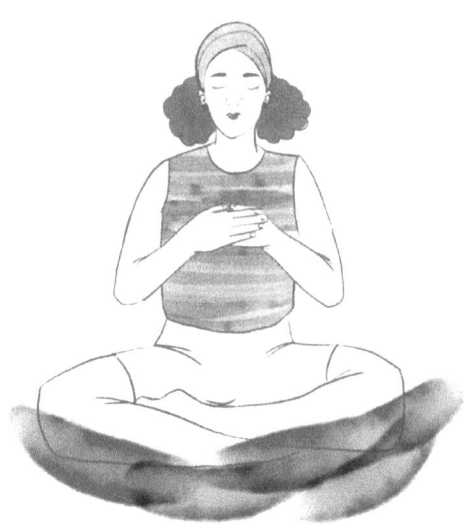

PART THREE
Remain in Easy Pose.

Mudra: Place the hands on the Heart Center, right on top of left.

Eye Focus: Tip of the Nose.

Breath: Not specified.

Mantra: Listen to the Sadhana mantras (Sangeet Kaur and Harjinder Singh's album *Raga Sadhana* was played in the original class.)

Time: 11 ½ minutes.

To End: Inhale deeply, suspend the breath for **15 seconds**, press hard on the Heart Center, squeeze the spine from bottom to top, and exhale. Repeat **2 more times**.

Comments: When you come from a place of love rather than fear, you become Karta (the lover), and then Prakriti (creation) provides everything you need.

*breathe, rest,
concentrate*

49 / **Be Yourself Meditation**

May 25, 1999

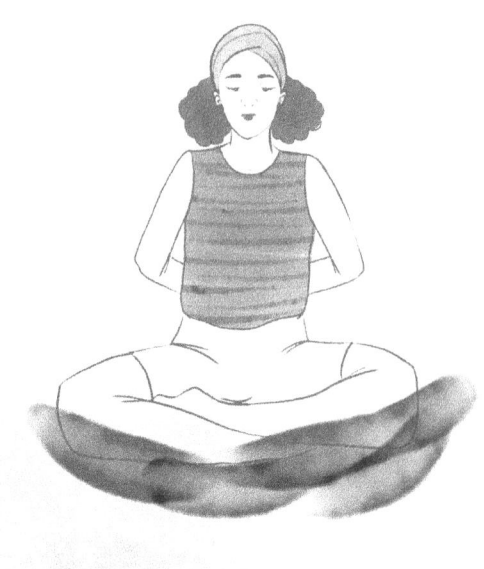

Sit in Easy Pose with a straight spine and a light Neck Lock.

Mudra: Interlock the hands at the base of the spine.

Eye Focus: 1/10th open and focused on the Tip of the Nose.

Breath: a) Inhale quickly and powerfully through the "O" mouth as you pull the diaphragm up and apply mulbandh in a jerking motion. Exhale quickly through the "O" mouth as you release the diaphragm and lock. Continue pumping the diaphragm strongly with the breath for **13 minutes.** b) Long Deep Breathing for **11 ½ minutes.** c) Breath of Fire for **3 minutes.**

Mantra: Listen to the recording "Hukam" by Singh Kaur and become thoughtless.

Total Time: 27 ½ minutes.

To End: Inhale deeply, suspend the breath for **15 seconds**, squeeze the body, move the diaphragm, and exhale. Repeat **2 more times.**

Comments: Life is made by our thoughts. Our subconscious collects unfulfilled thoughts, and when it gets full, thoughts overflow into the conscious mind. When this happens, we can react by isolating ourselves, not really listening, attempting to control everything, or doing nothing. With a disciplined meditation practice, we can empty the subconscious and filter those thoughts that get through to the conscious mind, choosing to attach to only the thoughts that serve and elevate us.

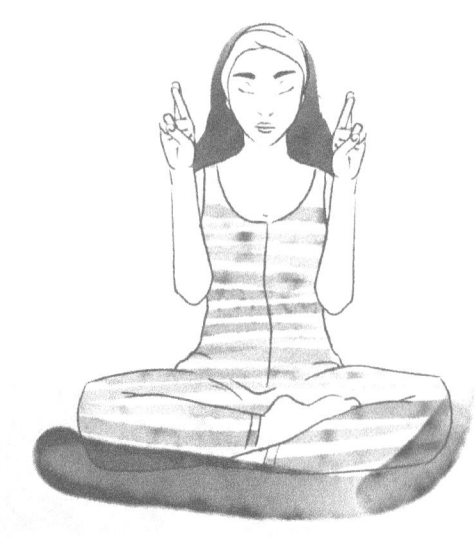

50 / **Kriya To Trust Yourself**

May 31, 1999

PART ONE
Sit in Easy Pose with a straight spine and a light Neck Lock.

Mudra: Raise the forearms up perpendicular to the ground with the elbows relaxed at the sides and the palms facing forward. Cross the Saturn (middle) fingers behind the Jupiter (index) fingers of both hands, keeping the other fingers upright.

Eye Focus: Not specified.

Breath: Long Deep Breathing through the "O" mouth, with the tip of the tongue pulled backward. Fill the lower abdomen completely with each breath.

Time: 20 minutes. Immediately begin Part Two.

PART TWO
Remain in Easy Pose.

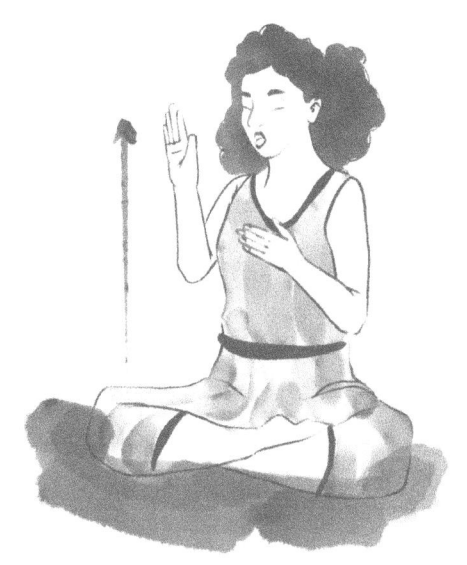

Mudra: Stretch the arms up with the hands facing forward and fingers stretched apart for the first **45 seconds**. Then try to lift the body off the ground by stretching the arms up for another **45 seconds**.

Eye Focus: Not specified.

Breath: Breath of Fire.

Time: 1 ½ minutes.

To End: Inhale deeply, stretch up and squeeze the entire body, suspend the breath for **15 seconds**, and exhale. Repeat **2 more times**.

Comments: When the kundalini, the dormant power in us, is awakened, we trust ourselves. We trust God, the Infinite. Our communication is clear, and our actions are trustworthy. We are seen for our dignity and divinity.

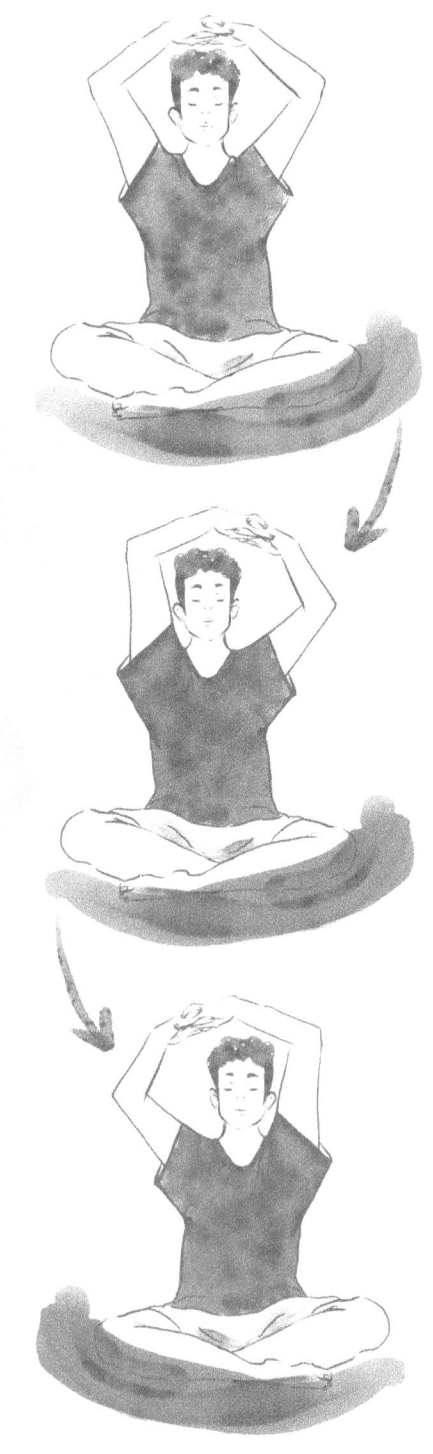

51 / **Know Yourself to Become a Leader**

June 1, 1999

Sit in Easy Pose with a straight spine and a light Neck Lock.

Mudra: Interlace the fingers and raise the arms to form an arc around the head with the palms facing down. Keeping the arms in an arc, inhale as you move the hands to the left, exhale, and return to the starting position. Inhale as you move the hands to the right, exhale, and return to the starting position. Move alternately at a pace of 5 times per second.

Eye Focus: Not specified.

Breath: Not specified.

Time: 20 ½ minutes.

To End: Inhale deeply, keeping the hands interlaced. Stretch the arms up, suspend the breath for **10 seconds**, and exhale. Repeat **1 more time.** Inhale deeply, place the hands on the Navel Point and press hard, suspend the breath for **10 seconds**, exhale, and relax.

Comments: In order to progress individually, we balance the tattvas (ether, air, fire, water, and earth) and the gunas (sattva, rajas, and tamas) within ourselves. Being in balance unveils our Divinity. Time and space will then serve us as we lead others.

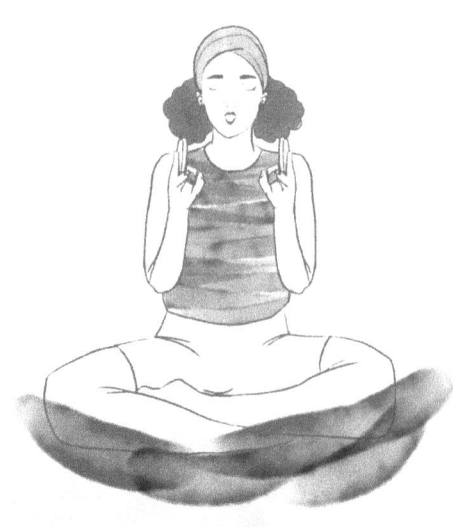

52 / Meditation to See All Life as a Blessing

June 7, 1999

Sit in Easy Pose with a straight spine and a light Neck Lock.

Mudra: Bring the hands in front of the shoulders in active Gyan mudra by locking the tip of the thumbs over the nails of the Jupiter (index) fingers and extending the other fingers straight up. The palms are facing each other.

Eye Focus: Tip of the Nose.

Breath: Long Deep Breathing through the "O" mouth. (The album "Meditate" by Singh Kaur was played in the original class.)

Time: 23 minutes.

To End: Inhale deeply, maintain the mudra and lips, suspend the breath for **15 seconds**, squeeze the body and the lips, push the energy to every fiber of the body, and exhale. Repeat **1 more time**. Interlace the fingers and stretch the arms up, inhale deeply, suspend the breath for **15 seconds**, and exhale.

Comments: There is only one creation, Ek Ong Kaar, and we are part of it. When we see the dualistic play of the universe as part of that one, the source solves our problems, and we see what it provides as an unequivocal blessing.

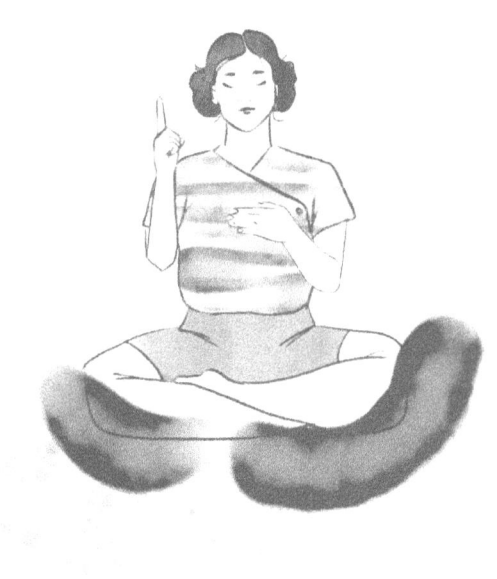

53 / **For a Golden Aura**

June 8, 1999

Sit in Easy Pose with a straight spine and a light Neck Lock.

Mudra: Place the left hand on the Heart Center. Bring the right hand by the shoulder with the palm facing to the left and the forearm perpendicular to the ground; extend the Jupiter (index) finger and hold the other fingers down with the thumb. Bring all the energy into the Jupiter (index) finger and keep it very stiff. Tighten the whole body for the last **30 seconds**.

Eye Focus: Tip of the Nose.

Breath: Cannon Breath.

Time: 18 minutes.

To End: Interlace the fingers and stretch the arms and spine up. Inhale deeply, suspend the breath for **20 seconds**, and exhale. Repeat **2 more times**.

Comments: When our aura is golden, we can help others, heal them, and calm them without touching them or saying a word. When we spend dedicated time with our innermost selves and develop balanced minds, our psyches and energy fields can give hope and comfort to others automatically.

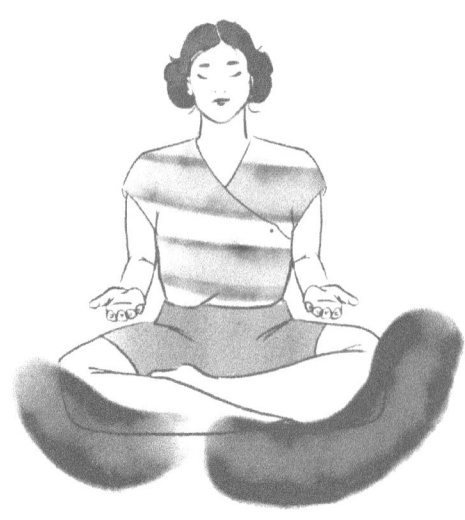

54 / **Face Yourself and Relax**

June 14, 1999

PART ONE
Sit in Easy Pose with a straight spine and a light Neck Lock.

Mudra: Press the elbows into the ribcage and bring the forearms forward parallel to the ground, with the palms facing up, hands cupped, and fingers relaxed apart.

Eye Focus: Tip of the Nose.

Breath: Inhale quickly and powerfully through the "O" mouth as you pull the diaphragm up in a jerking motion. Exhale quickly and powerfully through the "O" mouth as you release the diaphragm. Continue for **14 minutes.** Close the eyes and continue with Long Deep Breathing for **7 minutes.**

Total Time: 21 minutes.

To End: Inhale deeply, suspend the breath for **10 seconds**, exhale. Repeat **1 more time**. Inhale deeply, suspend the breath for **20 seconds**, and stretch the body. Immediately begin Part Two.

PART TWO

Remain in the posture. Continue to stretch and relax every part of the body.

Eye Focus: Not specified.

Breath: Not specified.

Time: 5 minutes. Immediately begin Part Three.

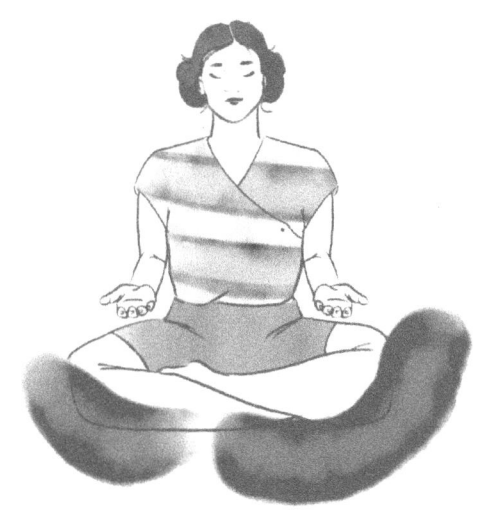

PART THREE

Sit in Easy Pose with a straight spine and light Neck Lock.

Mudra: Stretch the arms straight forward with the palms facing down. Rapidly move the arms a few inches (8-10 cm) up and down, as if bouncing a ball, keeping the arms straight. Move as quickly as possible (16 times per second).

Eye Focus: Not specified.

Breath: Not specified.

Time: 1 ½ minutes.

Comments: When we are afraid to face life, we lie to ourselves. Maintaining this false sense of who

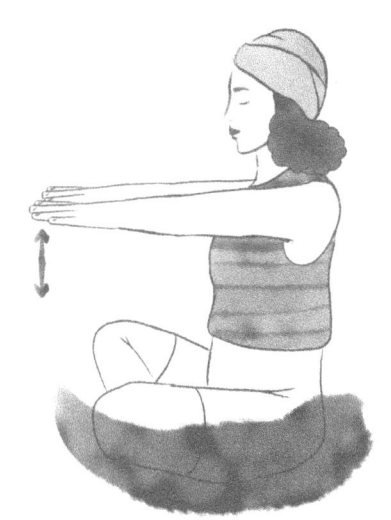

CONTINUE ON NEXT PAGE »

we are, we are unable to relax; we seek relaxation through external stimulation such as alcohol and drugs. Alternatively, when we raise the kundalini, it is like a light that illuminates the darkest corners of ourselves. Through practice, the nervous system is strengthened, and we build our capacity to be present in the discomfort. Facing our reality, we can relax in our truth. In this state, we experience Ang Sang Wha-hay Guroo and see God in ourselves and others.

breathe, rest, concentrate

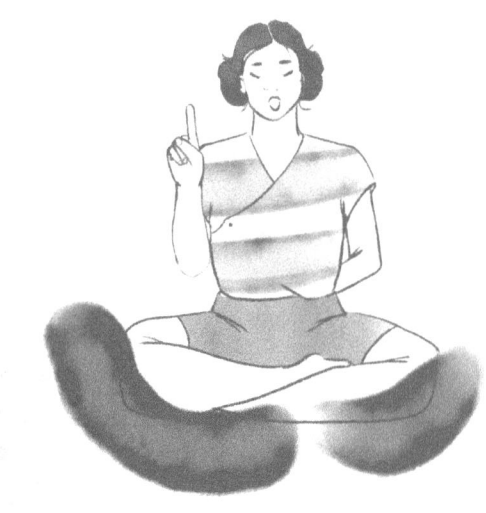

55 / **Know Yourself and Conduct Yourself**

June 15, 1999

PART ONE
Sit in Easy Pose with a straight spine and a light Neck Lock.

Mudra: Place the left hand on the lower spine with the palm facing out. Extend the right Jupiter (index) finger and hold the other fingers down with the thumb. Bring the right hand by the shoulder with the palm facing forward and the elbow by the side.

Eye Focus: 1/10th open.

Breath: Inhale quickly and powerfully through the "O" mouth as you pull the diaphragm up in a jerking motion. Exhale quickly and powerfully through the "O" mouth as you release the diaphragm.

Time: 19 minutes.

To End: Inhale deeply, exhale, and immediately begin Part Two.

PART TWO
Remain in Easy Pose.

Mudra: Place the hands on the Heart Center, right on top of the left.

Eye Focus: 1/10th open.

Breath and Mantra: Long Deep Breathing for **2 minutes**. Chant the Siri Gaitri Mantra **RAA MAA DAA SAA, SAA SAY SO HUNG** from the heart for **5 minutes**. (The Pachelbel's Canon version was played in the original class.)

Total Time: 7 minutes.

To End: Inhale deeply, suspend the breath for **15 seconds**, tighten and vigorously move the body, consciously sending energy to the whole body, and exhale. Repeat **2 more times.**

Comments: There is nothing to know but ourselves, for everything is within us. When we know ourselves, including our dark shadows, we can conduct ourselves through challenges by changing gears when necessary, pacing ourselves, managing our emotions, being authentic, and knowing which path to take. When we are committed to our higher selves, we apply our purity in all dealings, and God loves the purity of our living authentic selves.

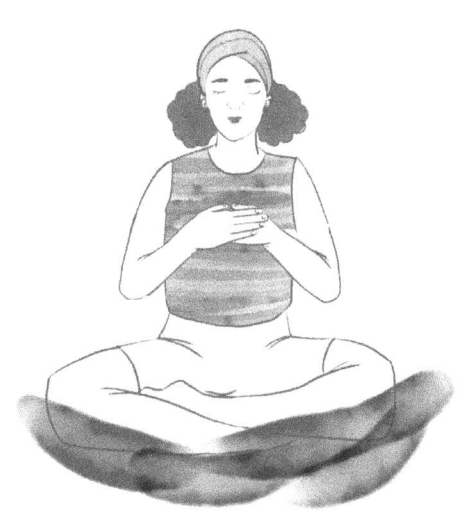

KRI is a non-profit organization that holds the teachings of Yogi Bhajan and provides accessible and relevant resources to teachers and students of Kundalini Yoga.

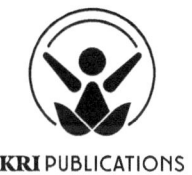

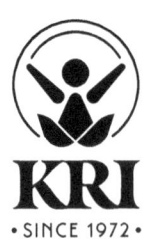

A Kundalini Yoga Global Community
KUNDALINIRESEARCHINSTITUTE.ORG

www.ingramcontent.com/pod-product-compliance
Lightning Source LLC
Chambersburg PA
CBHW040006040426
42337CB00033B/5237